—— **THE** ——

BAKING
SODA

COMPANION

ALSO BY SUZY SCHERR:

The Apple Cider Vinegar Companion

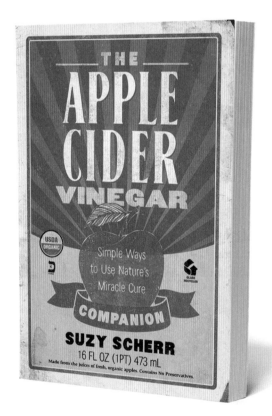

THE
BAKING
SODA
COMPANION

Natural Recipes and Remedies
for Health, Beauty, and Home

SUZY SCHERR

The Countryman Press
A division of W. W. Norton & Company
Independent Publishers Since 1923

For information about special discounts for bulk purchases, please contact
W. W. Norton Special Sales at specialsales@wwnorton.com or 800-233-4830

Manufacturing by Versa Press
Book design by Faceout Studio
Production manager: Lauren Abbate

The Countryman Press
www.countrymanpress.com

A division of W. W. Norton & Company, Inc.

500 Fifth Avenue, New York, NY 10110
www.wwnorton.com

978-1-68268-184-8 (pbk.)

10 9 8 7 6 5 4 3 2

For my family. Always.

CONTENTS

OUTDOOR USES FOR BAKING SODA 163

10 FUN THINGS TO DO WITH BAKING SODA 189

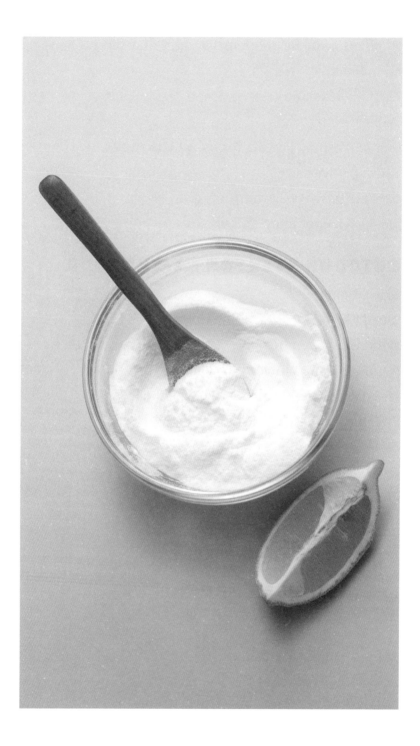

INTRODUCTION

You know those people who make it all look easy? Life: working, maintaining a social life, and maybe even taking care of kids, pets, or . . . (dare I say it?) plants. I'm not one of *those* people. I don't juggle it all with ease. I think it's hard to do all of those things at the same time! (Especially the plants part. I am a shamefully negligent plant parent.) Sure, there are days when I'm just *killing* it! Work is good: I'm cranking out great recipes for happy clients; I've posted something pretty and delicious on social media; and my inbox is clear of unanswered emails. The headquarters are in order: laundry is done; dinner is made; bathrooms are clean; and I'm wearing makeup *and* clean clothes. But then there are days—most days—when I need all the help I can get. To that end, I rely on an arsenal of shortcuts, hacks, and secret weapons to keep my crew healthy and well fed, my home clean and welcoming, and myself looking presentable (and sane). Enter: baking soda, my genie in the bottle—or, rather, in the cardboard box.

It is KFC's original recipe. It's Coca-Cola Classic. Baking soda has been around forever and is the miracle product you already own, but probably don't use to its full potential. It may make your fridge smell better, but that's just the tip of the icebox (hee hee). I'm convinced that a box of baking soda will solve just about any problem you might possibly encounter around the house. For pennies an ounce, baking soda can replace dozens of products. It naturally cleans the shower, refreshes carpets, washes dishes, destroys mold, and removes stains. I use it to wash my hair, make deodorant, take the *blech* out of sweaty gym clothes, soothe indigestion, and polish silver. (Hahahaha. I don't really polish silver. But *you* could. And then you could tell me how you found the time . . .) Baking soda is one of the best face exfoliators I've ever used; it's like micro-dermabrasion. And, of course, it makes its way into muffins and breads, but it also shows up in my super-fluffy omelets and as a surprise ingredient in my weeknight tomato sauce. Plus it's great for art projects, crafting, and DIY science experiments; so really, you can even entertain kids with it. Talk about multitasking!

As much as I would love to take credit as the Baking Soda Pioneer, as with my previous apple cider vinegar obsession, baking soda's age-old street cred has allowed it to maintain a cult following since pretty much the beginning of time. Ancient Egyptians were the first ones to use it as a kind of soap and people have enjoyed its versatility ever since. Amazingly, it took more than 100 tons of baking soda to clean the Statue of Liberty during its 1986 restoration! Your grandma's grandma probably knew of about six uses for baking soda around the home. So, what makes it so special that we can eat it but also clean our socks with it? Beyond being a good leavening agent, baking soda, a.k.a. sodium bicarbonate, is actually a salt. (Taste it and you'll see what I mean.) It acts like a cleaning agent because it is mildly alkaline (the opposite of acidic), making dirt and grease dissolve easily in water. That very alkaline nature is also what allows baking soda to neutralize odors, which are mostly acidic. It is slightly abrasive, so when sprinkled on a damp sponge, for example, it acts as a scouring powder, albeit one that's gentle, safe, and effective enough for delicate surfaces, such as glass, chrome, steel, enamel, and plastic. Because it is a pure, natural product that is also a food, it is nontoxic—unlike many other household and beauty products—so it's green and safe to use around children and pets.

So, get that box out from behind the container of Tuesday night's meatballs and experience firsthand this tried-and-true workhorse. Amidst the chaos of life, I use baking soda every single day to save time (and sanity) so that I can enjoy my kids, my family, and my friends. And so can you.

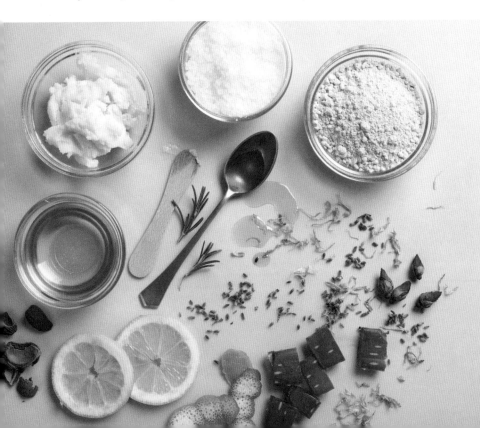

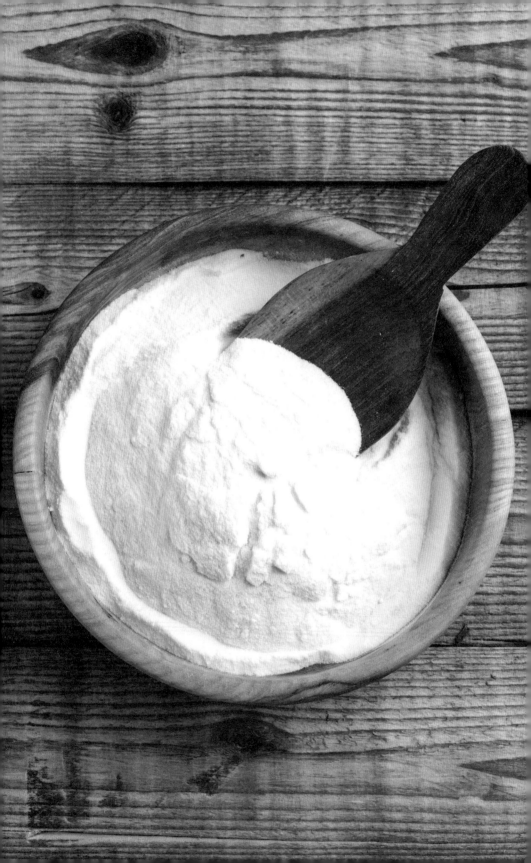

Change by:

/ / /

MONTH / DAY / YEAR

Write the date that is 30 days
from opening this box above.

FREE

**TABLESPOON
INSIDE**

PART ONE

THE ABCs
OF
BAKING SODA

Do n
bee
sig
O

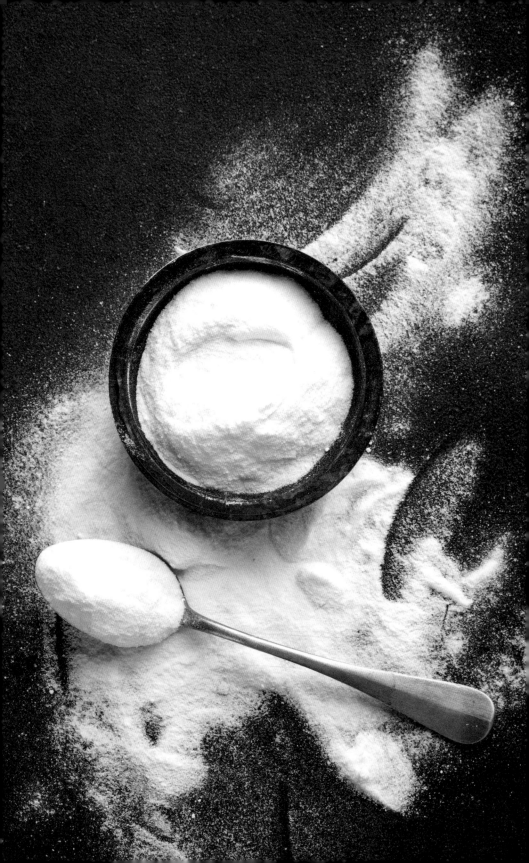

Everyone Knows Baking Soda, but—Seriously—What *Is* It?

The short answer: It's ground-up rock. In "geek speak," that means it is a chemical compound with the formula $NaHCO_3$. Baking soda—a.k.a. bicarbonate of soda, a.k.a. sodium bicarbonate—originates from one of two white or colorless minerals, either of which can be processed into what we all know as baking soda. A small percentage of the world's baking soda supply comes from a natural mineral called nahcolite, the majority of which is found in large quantities in Searles Lake, California, and the oil-shale deposits of Green River Formation in Colorado. But the rest (about 90 percent, actually) of the earth's baking soda comes from a natural mineral ore called trona, which is a gray, white, or yellowish mineral (I know this because I did a Google image search and I've got to tell you, trona crystals are pretty! I'd wear trona earrings. I'm just saying . . .). Trona is largely mined in Wyoming by Church and Dwight Company, makers of Arm and Hammer Baking Soda. According to the U.S. Geological Survey, Wyoming alone contains 56 million tons of pure trona (plus another 47 billion tons of trona that's been mixed with other minerals). Because we only mine about 15 million tons of trona per year (?!), the Wyoming Mining Association estimates that we have enough on hand to last us a couple thousand years. So . . . yeah, I think we're good.

Of course, to get from raw mineral ore to indispensable household staple requires a bit of a journey. Trona must first be extracted from the earth, then refined in a purification process that involves crushing the ore, heating it to drive off unwanted gases, and ultimately producing something called soda ash or sodium carbonate. That substance is then further processed through a multistep method of carbonation, centrifuges, driers, and some very cool chemistry that results in baking soda as we know it.

How Does It Work and What Can It Do?

Molecularly speaking, baking soda has a crystalline structure, which makes it somewhat abrasive; because it's water soluble, however, when baking soda gets wet, the edges of those crystals partially soften and dissolve before they can scratch or damage a surface. This is one of the reasons baking soda is such a fabulous cleaner: It's gentle but strong. Kind of like Mary Poppins.

It's also an acid neutralizer. Think back to high school chemistry class for a moment. (If you smiled just now, good for you! I, unfortunately, cringe instantly as I recall an extremely embarrassing mishap involving a Bunsen burner and an exploding test tube, but I digress . . .) Remember learning about the pH scale? It runs from 1 to 14, with 1 being a strong acid and 14 being a strong base (alkali). Baking soda has a pH of about 8, so it is a mild alkali. When combined with an acid, baking soda can bring a pH almost to neutral, which comes in handy in a ton of everyday scenarios, such as calming an upset stomach, covering up a bad smell, or relieving an itchy

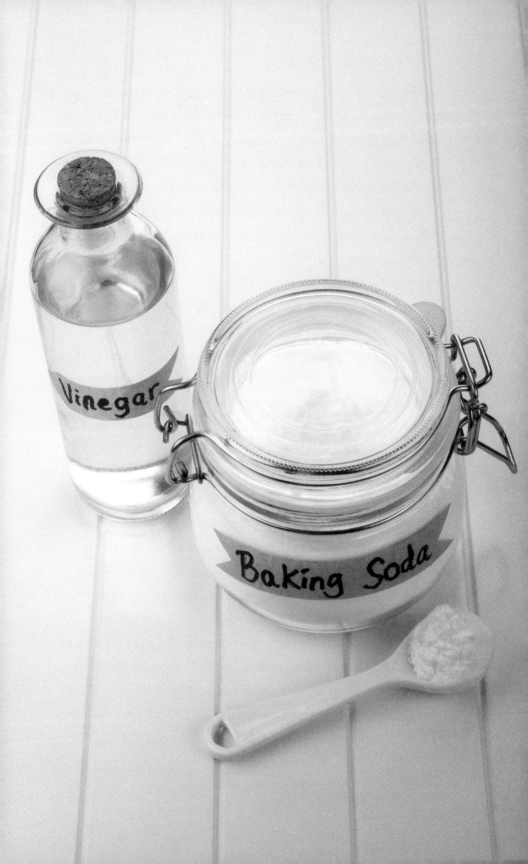

bug bite. But it's also becoming increasingly important in helping to treat some major diseases. While no studies have yet found that baking soda cures cancer, they have shown that some cancer treatments and chemotherapy drugs work better in alkaline environments. This means that baking soda, with its neutral pH, can create an ideal environment in a patient's body. Other studies have shown that patients with chronic kidney diseases, who took baking soda orally in conjunction with regular treatments, experienced a significantly slower kidney decline. That's likely because when kidneys don't work properly, they can't remove acid from the bloodstream. Adding baking soda to the mix neutralizes the blood, reducing the strain on already taxed kidneys. Pretty cool.

Of course, baking soda is best known for its mad skills as a leavening agent. It is so commonplace nowadays to use it in baking that it's hard to imagine a time when cooks could *only* rely on lengthy kneading processes and/or yeast to make baked goods rise. It really wasn't until the mid-1800s that baking soda became commercially available to home cooks. Since then, the handy dandy acid-based chemical reaction we know and love has been helping bakers around the world turn out quick breads, muffins, cakes, and cookies in a fraction of the time. And here's how: When baking soda—which we know is an alkali—is added to a batter or dough with an acid, such as vinegar, lemon juice, buttermilk, yogurt, or even chocolate, it produces carbon dioxide gas bubbles. Those small bubbles become trapped in batter, causing it to inflate, or rise.

Buying and Storing Baking Soda

I am here to tell you that baking soda is baking soda is baking soda. Finally, a product you just can't get wrong. Buy whatever brand you like, pick the box that looks cutest on your countertop, use what your grandmother used, get the one that's on sale. Honestly, thankfully, it doesn't really matter, because it's all pretty much the same stuff. Such a relief, right?

And as far as storing it, baking soda has an extremely long shelf life. It can't just suddenly "go bad." But, you should, ideally, store baking soda in a cool, dry place. Prolonged exposure to extreme heat, any temperature over 120°F, can definitely damage baking soda, but unless you live at the base of a volcano or . . . oh, I don't know . . . in the Sahara Desert, I think you can safely assume that your box of baking soda will stay good indefinitely. You may want to store it in an airtight container for moisture's sake, but even an opened cardboard box stays just fine for a good long time. So, keep it dry, keep it cool-ish, and you're all set. But do promise me this: The box that you have in your fridge to absorb odors stays in the fridge. OK? You leave that one there and go buy yourself another box for cooking and baking. You don't want to eat that smelly fridge baking soda. Gross. Promise!

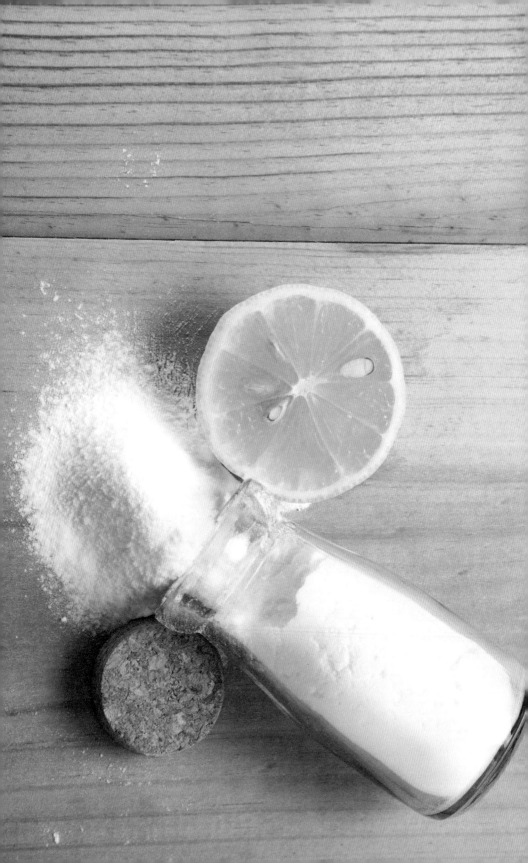

PART TWO

CLEVER WAYS TO USE BAKING SODA AT HOME

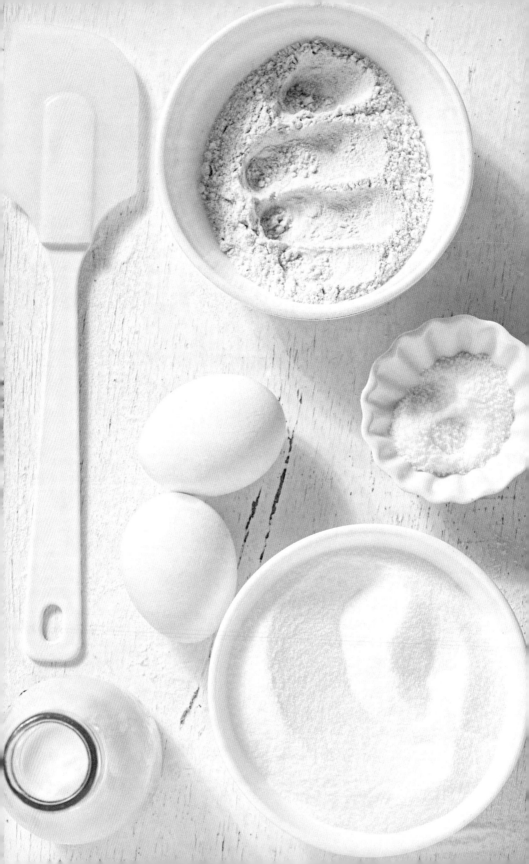

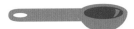

KITCHEN TRICKS AND HACKS

Baking soda originated in the kitchen and is, obviously, indispensable when it comes to baking—but it's a much more versatile cooking ingredient than you might think. Not only is it the secret to making authentic-tasting soft pretzels, crispy roasted potatoes, and the quickest-ever caramelized onions, but because of its chemical makeup, in a pinch (get it?), baking soda can correct too-sour or too-bitter flavors in food. Here are a few of my favorite baking soda hacks that magically make food crispier, chewier, fluffier, smoother, clearer, faster . . . better.

THE FLUFFIEST SCRAMBLED EGGS. EVER.

Eggs are so often the answer in our house. It's a busy weeknight, I never made it to the grocery store, and I have to get dinner on the table pronto. What's it gonna be? Eggs. Or, it's a rainy Sunday morning, we slept late, and now we want to eat a satisfying breakfast while lingering in our jammies for longer than I'd care to admit. Again, eggs. They're cheap, low in calories, easy to cook, and filled with a lot of nutrients that are otherwise difficult to find: the full spectrum of B vitamins, omega 3s, zinc, copper, and more. But they have to be done right, because bad eggs are about as big a bummer on a plate as I can think of. Perfect scrambled eggs, by my definition, are meltingly soft and fluffy, almost like a cloud. To get them that way, I use baking soda, which reacts with the eggs' natural acidity and creates pillowy air pockets.

Serves 4

8 large eggs
Kosher salt and pepper to taste
1 tablespoon unsalted butter
½ teaspoon baking soda

1. In a medium bowl, whisk the eggs and baking soda with a pinch of salt and a grind or two of black pepper until light and frothy.

Continued

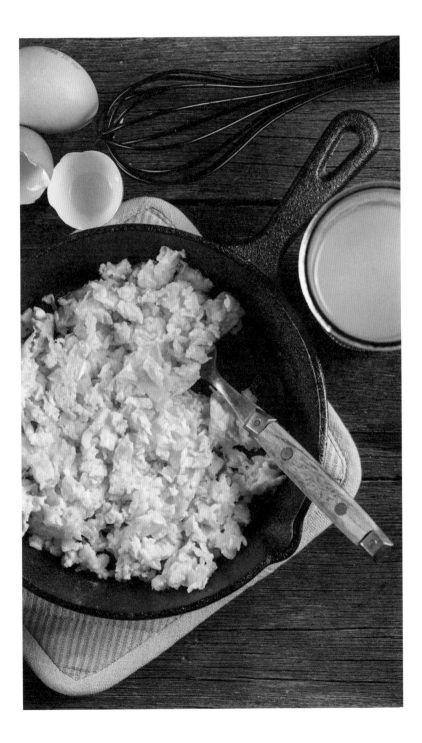

2. Melt the butter in a 10- or 12-inch nonstick skillet over medium-low heat.

3. Add the beaten eggs to the pan and stir slowly with a wooden spoon or spatula, bringing in all the beaten egg from the edges of the pan to the center, forming large curds.

4. Your eggs are ready when they look just a teensy bit under-cooked and still slightly runny—they'll continue to cook slightly even after you've removed them from the heat.

5. Serve immediately.

SOFT PRETZELS

More than just the shape, what makes a pretzel a pretzel is the quick dip it takes in an alkaline bath before hitting the oven. Without it, you'd be looking at an awfully bland, twisted dinner roll, since pretzels are more or less white bread at birth. The baking soda spa treatment gives pretzels their signature chewy crust and their unique pretzel flavor. Real-deal pretzels are bathed in food-grade lye, but that can be difficult to get your hands on and, frankly, not worth the risk, since it's a hazardous chemical that requires special safety measures in order to use it correctly. The good news is that baking soda makes an excellent substitute—it's the method I use to get dark, chewy pretzels at home. Go ahead and make a batch of your favorite recipe for sandwich bread dough (or pretzel dough for that matter) or, for a super speedy approach, follow these instructions for making darn good pretzels with ready-to-bake pizza dough.

Makes 6 to 8 large pretzels

1 (1-pound) ball pizza dough (see tip)
3 tablespoons baking soda
1 large egg
1 teaspoon water
Coarse salt for sprinkling

1. Preheat oven to 450°F.

2. Line two large baking sheets with parchment paper or greased foil.

Continued

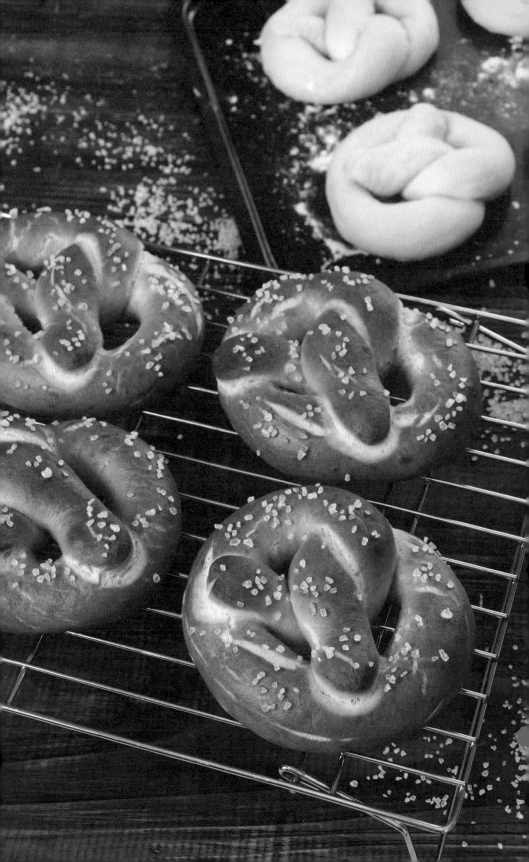

3. Divide the pizza dough evenly into 6 or 8 pieces, depending on how large you want your pretzels. Roll each piece into a long rope, about 20 inches. Pick up the ends of the rope and cross them. Cross them one more time to make a twist, then fold the twist back down over the bottom of the loop you've just made to form a pretzel shape.

4. In a wide saucepan or Dutch oven, bring 6 cups of water to a boil and add baking soda. Working with 2 pretzels at a time, boil for 30 seconds, then flip the pretzels over and boil for another 30 seconds. Remove them from the water using a slotted spoon, and place onto the prepared baking sheet. Repeat with the remaining dough.

5. Whisk the egg with one teaspoon of water in a small bowl. Brush the pretzels with the egg wash, then sprinkle with coarse salt.

6. Bake until golden brown, 11 to 12 minutes.

Tip: Hit up your local pizzeria and ask to buy uncooked dough.

DREAMY, CRISPY ROASTED POTATOES

I believe it to be more fact than opinion that perfectly roasted potatoes—golden brown, crispy yet somehow also creamy—are supreme. Making decent and even good roasted potatoes isn't difficult. After all, it's as simple as cutting up some potatoes, tossing them in oil and salt, then roasting them in a hot oven until golden. But making *seriously delicious* roasted potatoes requires one extra step that makes all the difference. The secret is boiling the potatoes in water that has been laced with baking soda before roasting them, which gives them unbelievably fluffy interiors. The baking soda bath breaks down the potato's pectin and draws the starch to the surface, which promotes browning and the satisfying crispiness that only a perfectly roasted potato can deliver. I like the flavor of Yukon gold, but feel free to substitute another potato variety.

Serves 4

2 pounds Yukon gold potatoes, peeled and cut into 1-inch dice

½ cup kosher salt

½ teaspoon baking soda

2 tablespoons extra virgin olive oil

¼ teaspoon pepper

Continued

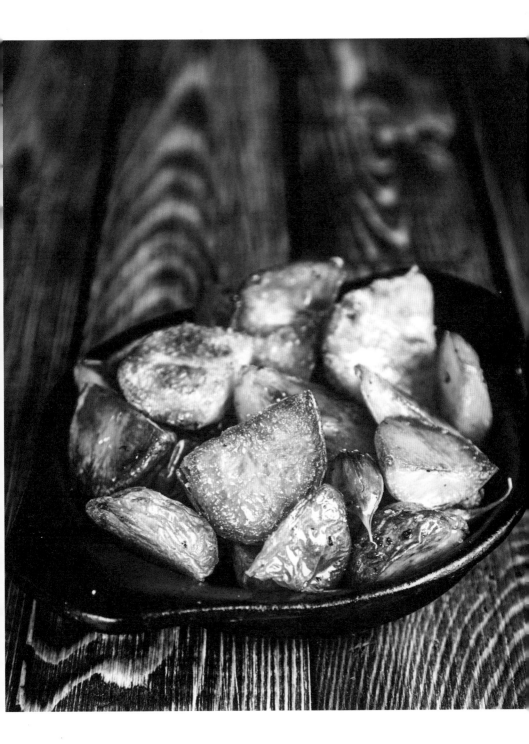

1. Place a large sheet pan in a cold oven, then preheat the oven to 500°F.

2. In a large pot, bring 8 cups water to boil. Add potatoes, salt, and baking soda. Return the pot to a boil, then reduce heat to simmer. Cook the potatoes for 5 minutes.

3. Drain the potatoes in a colander and shake vigorously to roughen edges. Transfer potatoes to a large bowl and toss with 1 tablespoon olive oil and pepper. Working quickly, carefully remove the sheet pan from the oven and pour the remaining 1 tablespoon oil onto the surface. Arrange the potatoes on the sheet in an even layer.

4. Bake until potatoes are crisp and skins are deep golden brown, about 20 to 25 minutes, stirring halfway through roasting.

5. Let cool on sheet for 5 minutes and serve.

SMOOTH-AS-SILK HUMMUS

You know that thick, grainy paste you scoop out of a plastic tub with baby carrots or pita chips when there's nothing else to eat in the fridge? That's not hummus. It may be called hummus, but believe me when I tell you that good hummus, real hummus, is something else entirely. It's fluffy, light, and unspeakably smooth. It isn't hard at all to make gorgeous, velvety hummus at home. It's really just a matter of cooking chickpeas, then blending them with garlic, lemon, tahini, and olive oil. Oh, but, according to droves of hummus experts, there's one teensy little thing you have to do to get it just right. You have to *peel* the chickpeas. Whuh? Um, yeah, you have to *peel* the chickpeas. I know it sounds time consuming and brain numbing. Yeah, because it IS! I know this, because when I first read about making perfectly smooth hummus this way at home, I had to try it—about halfway through peeling my 4 zillionth chickpea I sort of lost my mind and had to ask my husband to take over. We both agreed that, while hummus made from scalped chickpeas was indeed pretty much perfection, we could live with merely acceptable homemade hummus. Perhaps someday we'd have a chance to travel again in the Middle East, which is where I had my first taste of hummus as it should be. But I'm impatient, so I did a bit of research to figure out if there were some way, ANY way around peeling those suckers and still end up with the hummus of my dreams. And wouldn't ya know it: Baking soda is the secret ingredient in amazing hummus! Cooking chickpeas with baking soda softens them—skin and all—yielding a much smoother, creamier finished product.

Continued

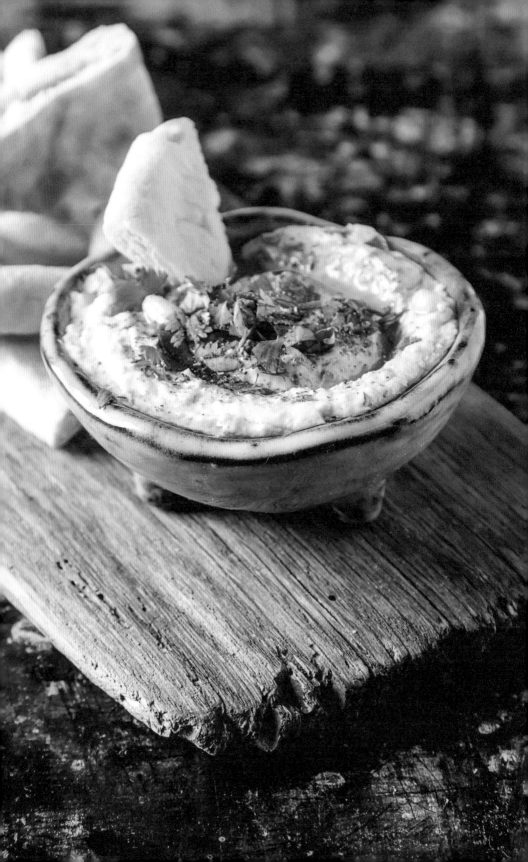

Makes about 2 cups

1 cup dried chickpeas

2 teaspoons baking soda

⅔ cup tahini

⅓ cup lemon juice

2 garlic cloves, peeled and crushed

1 teaspoon kosher salt

¼ cup ice water

Extra virgin olive oil (for serving)

1. Place chickpeas and 1 teaspoon baking soda in a medium bowl. Add enough cold water to cover by 2 inches. Cover and leave on the counter to soak overnight. Drain and rinse.

2. Combine soaked chickpeas and remaining teaspoon of baking soda in a large saucepan and cover with 2 inches of cold water. Bring to a boil, skimming loose skins from the surface as needed. Reduce the heat to medium-low, cover partially, and simmer until chickpeas are very soft and falling apart, about 45 to 60 minutes. Drain.

3. Place the chickpeas in a food processor and blend until smooth. With the machine running, add the tahini, lemon juice, garlic, and salt. Slowly add in the ice water and allow it to mix for about five minutes, until you achieve a very smooth, creamy mixture.

4. To serve, spoon hummus into a shallow bowl, drizzle liberally with oil.

PERFECT SHRIMP

Shrimp is a tasty and healthy delicacy that can be the show-piece of a delicious and satisfying meal. Or, as Bubba shrimp aficionado of *Forrest Gump* fame so eloquently explains:

> *. . . shrimp is the fruit of the sea. You can barbecue it, boil it, broil it, bake it, sauté it. There's, uh, shrimp-kabobs, shrimp Creole, shrimp gumbo. Pan-fried, deep fried, stir-fried. There's pine-apple shrimp, lemon shrimp, coconut shrimp, pepper shrimp, shrimp soup, shrimp stew, shrimp salad, shrimp and potatoes, shrimp burger, shrimp sandwich. That—that's about it.*

So there you have it: the definitive list of shrimp recipes. (*Wink.*) The bottom line is People Love Shrimp. But there is one tricky thing about them: They can quickly overcook. So if you're going to make shrimp, use this trick to ensure that they're plump, juicy, and firm, no matter how you're preparing them. Because nobody likes rubbery shrimp!

Serves 2 to 4

1 teaspoon kosher salt
¼ teaspoon baking soda
1 pound shrimp, peeled and deveined

1. Add salt, baking soda, and shrimp to a bowl. Toss to combine.

2. Cover and refrigerate for 15 to 45 minutes.

3. Cook as desired.

HOOKED ON SHRIMP

The method above prepares shrimp (fresh or frozen) to be added to any recipe that calls for them. If you don't have a recipe in mind, here are three quick ways to turn brined shrimp into dinner.

To roast shrimp: Toss 1 pound brined shrimp with 1 minced garlic clove, 2 teaspoons extra virgin olive oil, ¼ teaspoon salt, and zest of 1 lemon. Arrange the shrimp in a single layer on a baking sheet and roast 6 to 8 minutes in a preheated 400°F oven, or until just opaque. Toss with lemon juice and any fresh herbs you happen to have on hand. Serve.

To sauté shrimp: Warm ¼ cup extra virgin olive oil in a large sauté pan over low heat. Add 3 thinly sliced garlic cloves and cook until they just begin to turn golden. Increase the heat to medium-high and add 1 pound brined shrimp, salt and pepper to taste, and any other seasonings you like. (For a Spanish-inspired dish, try 1 teaspoon cumin and 1 teaspoon smoked paprika.) Toss to combine. Cook, stirring occasionally, just until the shrimp are pink all over, approximately 5 to 7 minutes. Remove from heat and toss with fresh parsley or other fresh herbs. Serve.

To grill shrimp: Make a quick marinade by combining ½ cup lemon or lime juice with ½ cup honey, 1 tablespoon extra virgin olive or vegetable oil, 2 minced garlic cloves, ½ teaspoon pepper, and 1 teaspoon salt. Place marinade and 1 pound brined shrimp into a bowl; toss to combine. Cover and refrigerate for 15 to 30 minutes (no longer or the citrus juice will "cook" the shrimp). Thread shrimp onto skewers or place in a grill basket. Place shrimp on a preheated grill and cook for 2 to 3 minutes per side, until just cooked. Remove from grill and serve.

SPEEDY CARAMELIZED ONIONS

For a busy cook, caramelized onions present a real quandary. Sure, they're deeply delicious, impossibly rich, meltingly savory... they're pure magic is what they are! But caramelizing onions is incredibly time consuming, requiring near-constant stirring for anywhere from 45 to 90 minutes. Not exactly busy weeknight fare. Or is it...? What if I told you it was possible to make savory-sweet, perfectly complex caramelized onions in as little as 15 to 20 minutes? You'd expect me and Doc Brown to take you for a ride in a DeLorean, to traverse the time-space continuum to the not-too-distant future, wouldn't you? Fun as that would be, time travel is not actually required to turn out amazing caramelized onions in a flash. Nope. But baking soda is. You see, just a pinch of baking soda increases the pH of onions, which speeds up something called the Maillard reaction, the process responsible for the browning of proteins in food. It can accelerate the browning rate by more than 50 percent! These onions, soft and sweet, are good on pretty much... everything. They keep for a week or more in the fridge, so it's fine to make them well ahead of time.

Makes about 1 cup

1 tablespoon unsalted butter

3 large yellow onions, peeled and sliced thin

¼ teaspoon sugar

⅛ teaspoon baking soda

Kosher salt and freshly ground black pepper

½ cup water

1. Melt butter in a large sauté pan over medium-high heat. Add onions, sugar, baking soda, and 1 teaspoon salt. Toss to combine. Cook, shaking and/or stirring the pan occasionally until onions begin to brown, about 6 to 8 minutes.

2. Deglaze the pan with 2 tablespoons of water, scraping with a wooden spoon to release all of the brown bits from the bottom of the pan. Cook for another 3 to 5 minutes, then deglaze again with another 2 tablespoons of water. Repeat a few more times until the onions are deeply browned and you've gone through the whole ½ cup of water.

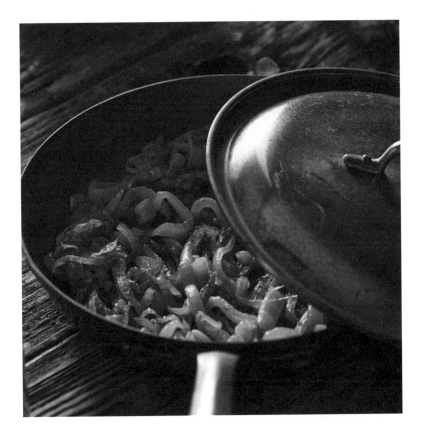

WEEKNIGHT TOMATO SAUCE

A few years ago we took our kids out to dinner at an Italian restaurant with another family. At the time, my eldest daughter was deep into a nothing-but-buttered-noodles phase (and, as such, I was deep into a trying-very-hard-not-to-scream-about-the-fact-that-I-am-a-professionally-trained-chef-and-why-are-you-doing-this-to-me phase). When it came time to order dinner, she, unsurprisingly, was not interested in wavering from her habit. That is, until our genius friend, Michelle, whispered in her ear, "You know, they have princess sauce at this restaurant. You could get a bowl on the side and dip your noodles." WHAT THE WHAT? "Princess sauce? I LOVE princess sauce!" said the little one. YOU LOVE IT? YOU DON'T EVEN KNOW WHAT IT IS! (Princess sauce = tomato sauce. I don't love using gimmicks to get kids to eat, but I'll take it.) Thus started a tomato sauce kick that is still going strong. I make it about once a week, using this dead easy, unbelievably delicious recipe that takes about as long to make as it does to cook pasta. FAST. Baking soda cuts the acidity (and occasional bitterness) without adding unnecessary sweetness, resulting in a perfectly balanced sauce that's, well . . . fit for royalty.

Makes about 2½ cups

1 (28-ounce) can crushed tomatoes

3 tablespoons unsalted butter

½ yellow onion, peeled

1 garlic clove, peeled

½ teaspoon kosher salt

⅛ teaspoon baking soda

1 sprig fresh basil (optional)

1. Add all ingredients to a medium saucepan and bring to a boil over medium-high heat.

2. Reduce the heat to medium-low and simmer for 15 to 20 minutes (or longer, if you have time).

3. Remove from the heat. Remove the onion, garlic, and basil, and discard.

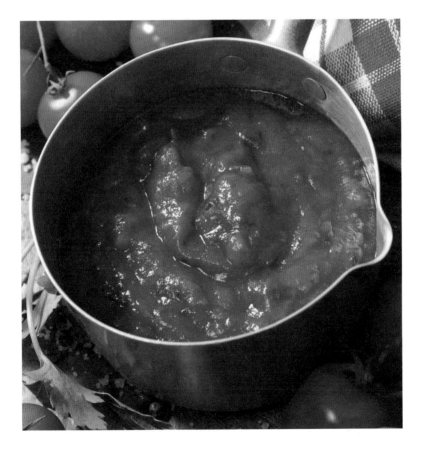

HOMEMADE RAMEN NOODLE HACK

Holy moly do I love ramen. And, by the way, I'm not talking about the "Peel off the lid. Pour boiling water into the cup. Let sit for three minutes. Stir well and serve" variety. I'm talking about huge bowls of chewy, luxurious noodles swimming in a flavorful, savory broth with an assortment of proteins, loads of garnishes, and a soft-boiled egg floating on top. Comfort food of the highest order. In winter (or anytime I'm not feeling well), nothing soothes quite like a bowl of ramen, but it's not always possible to get my hands on the real McCoy. And while making flavorful Japanese-inspired soup at home isn't difficult, subbing in regular pasta for ramen noodles just doesn't do the dish justice. Ramen noodles have a springier, stronger texture than other styles of pasta and a distinct savory taste in the dough that comes from an alkaline element known as *kansui*. It isn't easy for most home cooks to find and—let's be honest—you're probably not going to make your own ramen noodles even if you could. BUT what other alkaline element do you love so very, very much because it can do absolutely anything, including making regular spaghetti look and taste a whole lot like authentic ramen noodles? BAKING SODA!!! (Sparkles! Rainbows! Yaaaay!) This hack is quick and satisfying. No Styrofoam cup required.

Serves 4

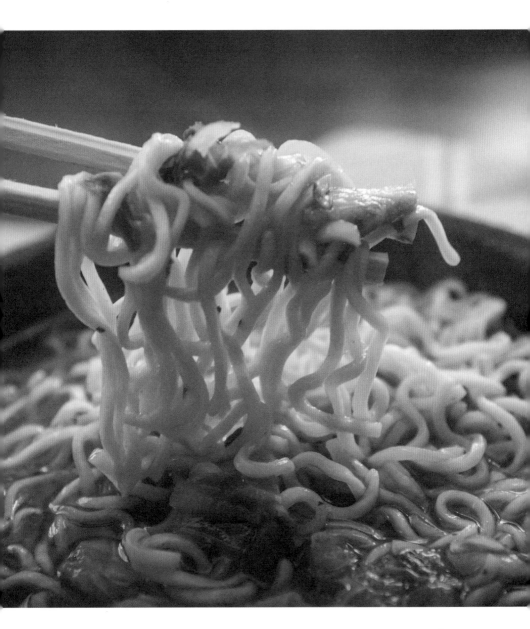

Continued

1 to 2 quarts water

1 to 2 tablespoons baking soda

1 pound spaghetti

1. Bring water to a boil in a large pot over high heat.

2. Slowly add 1 tablespoon of baking soda for each quart of water. The water will still bubble and foam, so make sure that you keep a close eye on it.

3. Add the spaghetti to the pot and cook 8 to 10 minutes, until al dente, springy, and yellow.

4. Drain, add to soup or broth of your choice, slurp, and enjoy.

ANATOMY OF A DELICIOUS AND VAGUELY AUTHENTIC (WEEKNIGHT) RAMEN BOWL

Noodles: spaghetti hacked with baking soda, as above

Nori: edible dried seaweed (the stuff that's on the outside of a sushi roll), shredded

Sliced scallions and spinach leaves: a handful of each

Soft-boiled eggs: cooked, peeled, and marinated in a bit of soy sauce, if you have time

Some kind of roasted or braised protein: shredded rotisserie chicken, roasted pork, cubed tofu, or ground meat

Soup base: miso, chicken, beef, pork—it all works

Other add-ins: a handful of corn kernels, a few dashes of hot sauce, sesame oil, sesame seeds, bamboo shoots, bean sprouts, Japanese pickles, shredded carrot, shredded cabbage, and/or mushrooms

DIY BAKING POWDER

We've all been there: You're headed to the kitchen to bake cookies and start to gather the ingredients when you suddenly realize that—d'oh!—you're all out of baking powder! Well, the next time you find yourself in a baking powder pinch, use this simple formula to make your own. Cream of tartar is an acidic powder, a byproduct from wine-making, and is commonly used as an egg white stabilizer in baking. Combining cream of tartar with baking soda takes no time at all to make ahead and stores almost indefinitely for whenever you need it, or when you need to whip it up last minute when a cookie emergency erupts.

Makes 3 tablespoons

1 tablespoon baking soda
2 tablespoons cream of tartar

1. In a small bowl, thoroughly whisk together baking soda and cream of tartar.

2. Store in an airtight, moisture-free container.

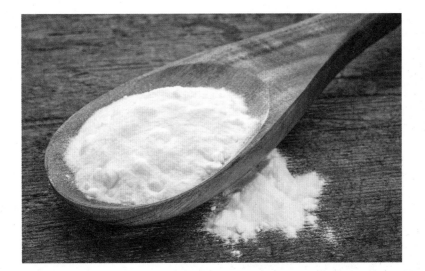

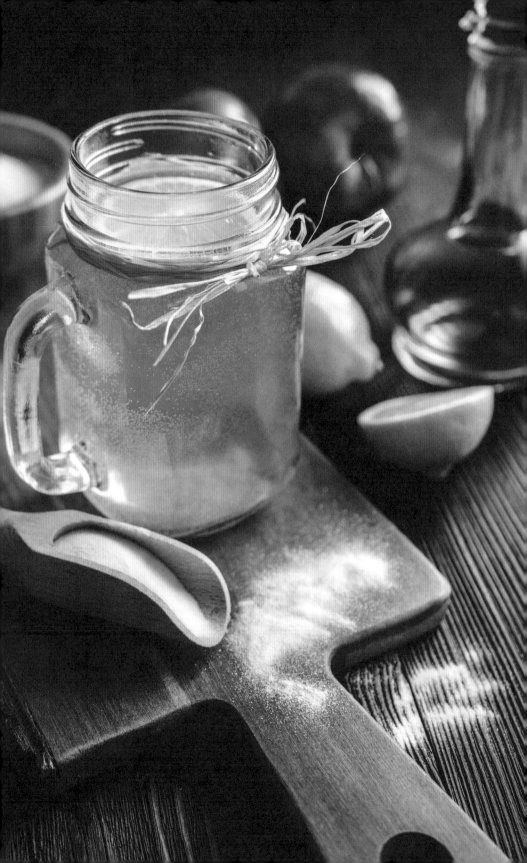

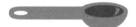

HEALING WITH
BAKING SODA

TUMMY TAMER

I think we can all agree that stomach pain is the worst. Heartburn, nausea, gas, indigestion—worst, worst, worst, worst. When things aren't right in the middle you can't sleep, you can't think, and you certainly can't eat. A bottle of antacid or other over-the-counter medicine can help, but it's just as easy to tame a troubled tummy naturally with sodium bicarbonate. And lest you think this is my idea, check the active ingredient on many over-the-counter antacid tablets and you'll find sodium bicarbonate right there in black and white, along with a bunch of other stuff you can't recognize or pronounce. Baking soda absorbs quickly into the intestines and neutralizes stomach acid, offering speedy relief. And the carbonation that occurs when it mixes with water promotes burping (only the most polite sort, I assure you), which relieves gas and bloating. Just remember: While baking soda is a superstar at taming stomach acid, there are tons of reasons why you might be encountering stomach pain; acid isn't the only one. If your symptoms don't improve after a week or so, check in with your doctor just to be sure you don't have something more serious going on.

For 1 use

¼ teaspoon baking soda
8 ounces water

Stir baking soda into a glass of water. Sip slowly.

Note: You shouldn't take baking soda within 2 hours of other medications. Because baking soda decreases stomach acid, it can slow down your body's absorption of some medicines and change the way others work. If you take medication, check with your doctor before drinking baking soda.

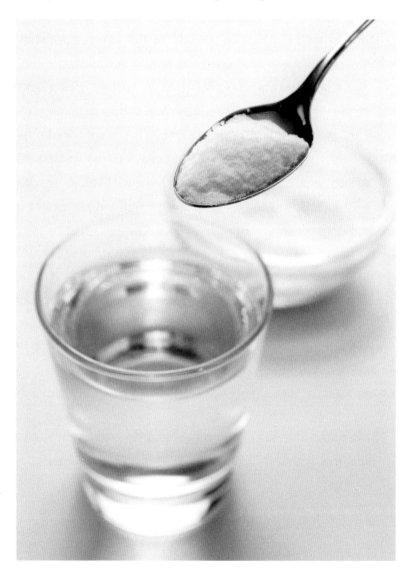

COLD AND FLU DETOX BATH

Being sick is a bummer for anyone, but being sick when you're a "real" grownup—as in, a person with a job and, y'know, RESPONSIBILITIES—is pretty abysmal. First of all, many of us grownups stink at being sick: We don't *really* rest and give ourselves time to heal, even though we all know it's probably what we ought to do. But work, meetings, social obligations, pets, kids, laundry, and other assorted "surprises" in our lives still require our superpowers, regardless of how high our temperature is or how miserable we feel. When a cold or the flu hits, everyone needs a quick fix to get back to life ASAP. This detox bath helps kick sick symptoms to the curb—baking soda and epsom salts rid the body of toxins, and ginger acts as a natural decongestant and pore opener. The combination gets that cold or flu over with quicker.

For 1 bath

1 to 2 cups Epsom salts
½ cup baking soda
4 tablespoons ground ginger
Essential oils of choice (optional)

1. Fill a bathtub with enough very warm water to completely submerge yourself—the hotter, the better (to promote sweating).

2. Sprinkle in Epsom salts, baking soda, ginger, and oils, if using. Stir.

3. Submerge yourself to your neck. Soak for 20 to 40 minutes.

4. Towel off, then rest for approximately 30 minutes (or as long as you can). Drink plenty of fluids before and after your detox bath.

Note: If you're pregnant or have heart or liver illness, you'll have to sit this one out. Instead, go ahead and wallow in your sickness. Get some magazines, binge on TV, and eat some rainbow sherbet. I won't tell.

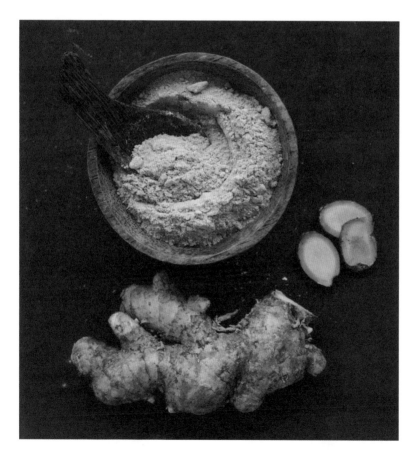

SINUS CLEANSE

Each year, as winter looms, I round everyone up for a fun-filled family outing to get flu shots. Once administered, I feel invincible, safe, and protected—it lasts about 20 minutes, until I remember that soon enough, the first round of whatever other lurking vaccine-less bugs out there will show up to infect my crew. This winter, when an ugly virus made its rounds, I was sick for about a day or two, but made a reasonably quick recov-

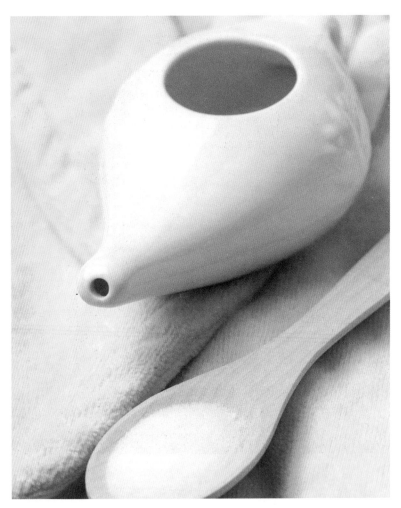

ery thanks to my own Cold and Flu Detox Bath (page 52). I soon felt like a person again, except for MY WHOLE ENTIRE HEAD, which felt like it had been filled in with cement. One side of my face was so swollen I looked like I'd been in the ring with Rocky Balboa. Fortunately, this sinus rinse provided quick relief so I could get back to wiping other people's noses.

For 1 use

¼ teaspoon non-iodized salt

¼ teaspoon baking soda

8 ounces lukewarm distilled (not tap) water

In a clean container, combine salt, baking soda, and water. Using a soft rubber ear bulb syringe, infant nasal bulb, or a nasal saline rinse product, such as a neti pot, use the rinse as follows:

1. Draw up saline into the bulb. Tilt your head downward over a sink (or in the shower) and rotate to the left. Squeeze approximately 4 ounces of solution gently into the right (top) nostril. Breathe normally through your mouth. In a few seconds, the solution should come out through your left nostril. Rotate your head and repeat the process on the left side.

2. Adjust your head position as needed so the solution does not go down the back of your throat or into your ears.

3. Blow your nose gently to prevent the solution from going into your ear, causing discomfort.

Caution: Do not use sinus rinse if your nasal passages are severely blocked.

SPLINTER REMOVER

I probably shouldn't need to be told that self surgery is rarely a good idea, and yet, for years, whenever I got a splinter my instant response was to set up what looked like an eighteenth-century operating room, save for the bottle of moonshine and the mason jar of leeches. I'd set out matches (for sterilizing, of course), needles, and tweezers, identify the approximate location of that tiny and surprisingly painful sliver of wood, glass, or whatever, then go about digging, scraping, and pulling until I yanked that sucker out. Except sometimes not. And either way . . . OW! Good news for the harebrained among us: Baking soda is a safe and effective way to remove splinters, especially the teensy ones you can feel but can't find.

For 1 use

¼ teaspoon baking soda
Water
Bandage

1. Clean the skin around the splinter, using soap and water.

2. Combine baking soda with enough water to give it a paste-like consistency.

3. Apply the paste to the cleaned area and put a bandage on top to keep it in place.

4. Leave the bandage on for 24 hours, and then remove. The splinter may be sticking out, in which case you can pull it out gently with tweezers. If you don't see it, repeat this process for another 24 hours, until you can grasp it with tweezers or feel that the splinter has worked its way out on its own.

ATHLETE'S FOOT TREATMENT

Surprising as it may be, you don't have to be an athlete to get athlete's foot. Anyone at all can wind up with the itchy-between-the-toes condition if two things happen: 1) their bare tootsies are exposed to *juuuust* the right kind of fungus; and 2) that fungus has *juuuust* the right environment in which to grow—such as in hot and sweaty gym shoes, for example. If you do end up with athlete's foot you'll most likely find that your feet and the skin between your toes will burn and itch like the Dickens. The skin may peel and crack. You will ~~want~~ need to find relief fast. And baking soda will be your knight in shining armor. Why? Because it balances the pH level of feet, creating an inhospitable environment for acid-loving fungus and bacteria. And bonus—it is an excellent exfoliant that softens the skin and removes the not-so-sporty calluses and peeled skin caused by athlete's foot. Here's how:

Baking Soda Foot Soak

For 1 use

2 to 4 liters water

3 tablespoons baking soda

1. Combine water and baking soda in a large bucket. Stir well to dissolve.

2. Soak feet in the baking soda water for 15 to 20 minutes, then use a clean scrub brush to clean your feet and in between your toes.

3. Wipe your feet with a clean towel and moisturize with coconut oil or petroleum jelly.

Baking Soda Rub

For 1 use

3 tablespoons baking soda
1 tablespoon water

1. Clean your feet thoroughly and pat dry with a towel.

2. Mix baking soda and water to form a thick paste.

3. Spread the paste evenly on your feet and in between your toes.

4. Let it dry on its own.

5. Rinse feet with cold water and pat dry with a towel.

EXERCISE-BOOSTING ELECTROLYTE DRINK

You know that nagging, dragging feeling you get when you're about halfway through an intense run, hike, spin class, or whatever it is you do for exercise? The feeling like you just. can't. anymore. There's a reason for that. See, our bodies are mostly made up of fluid, which means that every cell plus all of our organs and tissue need enough water to do their jobs. When you sweat buckets in a booty-popping, hip-shaking jazzercise class, you deplete the supply. This is what makes you feel like taking a nap on the Zumba floor. While plain water is the most important part of hydration, we also lose electrolytes (e.g. potassium and sodium) when we sweat and we need those in order for nerve impulses and muscle contractions to work properly. This performance-boosting, all-natural, no-artificial-junk tonic, with electrolytes in the form of sea salt and baking soda, will not only hydrate you, it'll help you go harder longer no matter what physical activity you're doing. This makes a big batch that you can swig over the course of a few days. Work it!

Makes 6 to 8 servings

½ teaspoon sea salt
¼ teaspoon baking soda
7 cups coconut water
½ cup lemon juice
¼ cup honey

1. Add all the ingredients to a large bottle or pitcher. Stir or shake to combine.

2. Store in the refrigerator for up to a week.

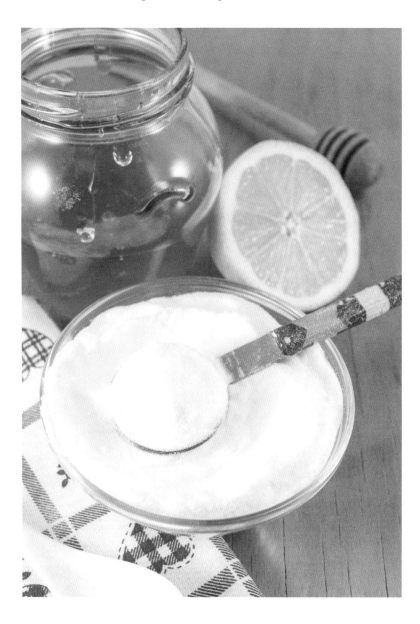

CONSTIPATION CURE

Hey, did you hear the one about the constipated composer? He couldn't finish the last movement! (Sorry.) There are a few possible causes for constipation—lack of fiber, inadequate fluids, and insufficient physical activity are chief among them. But if you've tried lifestyle tweaks and are still backed up, consider turning to baking soda. It reacts with stomach acids to cleanse the colon and treat constipation. Because it's a salt, baking soda draws fluids into the gastrointestinal tract, causing a series of wave-like muscle contractions that move food through the intestines. It is also a mild laxative, loosening bulky stools, thus making it less painful to go number two. Try it and soon enough the only groan you'll release is at the end of this joke: Did you hear about the constipated *Wheel of Fortune* contestant? She needed to buy a bowel. (Sorry again.)

For 1 use

1 teaspoon baking soda
¼ cup lukewarm water
Pinch of salt

1. Combine all the ingredients in a glass. Stir to dissolve.

2. Drink on an empty stomach, ideally, first thing in the morning.

Note: If your constipation doesn't respond to changes in diet, lifestyle changes, or home remedies, it's time to see your doctor.

BURN TREATMENT

Want to know what doesn't feel great? Brushing your arm against the edge of a 500°F oven or finding yourself on the wrong side of some splattering duck fat. Take it from me: If you spend enough time in a kitchen, you're going to get burned. Professional cooks, especially those working on a busy line, have no choice but to tough it out through the pain as they bang out their orders. They don't ditch the dinner service to dab on antibiotic ointment and cuddle an ice pack. Occupational hazard or not, I'll admit: burns hurt and I've turned to baking soda plenty to soothe the angry pain. This remedy works on all kinds of burns—even sunburns—offering quick and lasting relief.

For 1 use

2 tablespoons baking soda
1 to 2 tablespoons cool water

1. Clean the affected area with cool water.

2. In a bowl, mix baking soda and water to make a paste.

3. Apply the mixture to the burn with a cotton ball. Leave for 5 to 10 minutes, then rinse with cool water.

4. Dry the skin thoroughly. Repeat as necessary.

FEVER-REDUCING BATH

I will confess to having overreacted to, over-treated, and over-thought fevers in my time on earth. When faced with a sick loved one, it's easy to forget that a fever in and of itself isn't *all* bad—it means a person's immune system is in working order, fighting an underlying infection or virus. Over time, I've learned to take a breath before acting on my first instinct to "fix" a fever with medicine as soon as I detect one, and instead try to remember that fever-reducing medicine will mask a fever, not cure it. (Once the meds wear off, a person's temp will soar back to triple digits if that's where you started, because the underlying cause is still there.) But anyone with a fever is a miserable, listless thing who just wants to feel better, so what can you do? The response to most fevers in our house is a good soak in a baking soda bath. It helps reduce a fever, making poor things regardless of age more comfortable and better able to rest.

For 1 use

1 cup baking soda

1. Fill a bathtub with enough warm water to submerge the body—water that is too hot can raise a fever and, counterintuitive as it may seem, so will water that is too cold, as it promotes shivering, which leads to a spike in fever.

2. Sprinkle in baking soda. Stir.

3. Submerge to the neck. Soak for 10 to 20 minutes.

CRADLE CAP ELIMINATOR

The onset of cradle cap is like something out of a 1950s classic horror film. Coming soon: Boris Karloff stars in *The Arrival of Cradle Cap*. Our film begins with a set of happy, new parents bringing a newborn home from the hospital, thoroughly positive that they've just birthed the most magnificent baby in history. They gaze adoringly, beaming with pride at this flawless, innocent little being. When all of a sudden [cue: menacing music] flakes and scales start popping up on their perfect child's scalp, occasionally spreading to the baby's face, clustering around the eyebrows. Oh no! It's here! It's . . . it's cradle cap!! Thankfully, cradle cap—the common term for seborrheic dermatitis—is actually a very common, non-contagious, non-infectious skin condition that will usually resolve on its own over time. It really bothers us parents more than our babies. Washing your baby's scalp daily with mild shampoo and using this home remedy can help to speed up the process of loosening and removing those scales caused by cradle cap.

For 1 use

1 teaspoon baking soda
1 teaspoon oil (such as olive, coconut, or almond)

1. Mix baking soda and oil to make a paste.

2. Gently massage into the baby's scalp, being very careful to avoid the eyes. Leave paste on for a few minutes.

3. Cleanse with a mild shampoo and water.

4. Repeat daily to eliminate cradle cap.

DIAPER RASH RELIEF

I once traveled on Amtrak from New York City to Washington, DC, with a rash-ridden six-month-old baby and realized somewhere near Wilmington, Delaware, that I'd left my tube of diaper rash cream at home in Brooklyn. I spent the next hour and a half simultaneously attempting to (and failing at) consoling a screaming baby while frantically Googling "instant diaper rash treatment," "fastest ways to treat diaper rash," and "tips for avoiding a nervous breakdown on mass transit." What I learned from search result after search result is that a diaper rash is acidic and baking soda is alkaline, so if I used it on my baby's irritated skin, it would neutralize the acidic nature of what was happening in her pants and help heal her sore tush. That night, desperate to relieve the poor, uncomfortable little thing who didn't seem to be getting any relief from the tube of seemingly too runny cream I'd hastily purchased at the train station newsstand, I dumped some baking soda in her bath water. I also mixed up a solution of baking soda and water in a spray bottle, which I stashed in the diaper bag. At every diaper change, I misted her, rinsing her well with clean water after each application, since baking soda can sting if it lingers too long on the skin. Sure enough, just as Dr. Google promised, in about a day and a half, her rash was healed and I was a convert.

Makes 2 cups

Continued

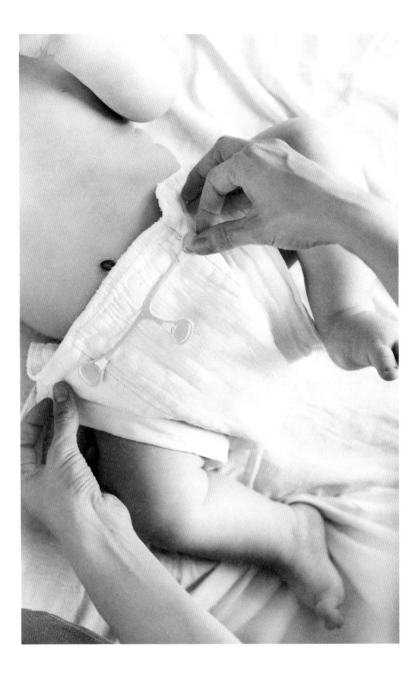

FOR SPRAY:

1 to 2 heaping tablespoons baking soda

2 cups warm water

1. In a clean spray bottle, mix baking soda and water.

2. With the bottle's nozzle set at the most gentle mist setting, lightly spritz baby's skin, being sure to completely wet the affected area.

3. Using a clean, wet cloth, a few cotton balls, or an unscented baby wipe, carefully wipe or pat the rash to thoroughly rinse the skin.

4. Diaper as usual.

FOR THERAPEUTIC BATH:

2 teaspoons baking soda

1. Add baking soda to a warm bath.

2. Bathe your baby for 10 to 15 minutes, then pat dry.

3. Repeat 2 to 3 times daily.

CANKER SORE RELIEF

If you suffer from canker sores, you know all too well that those little suckers can cause major mouth pain. You might get them on the inside of your lip or cheek, under your tongue, or at the base of your gums. Sometimes they're even audacious enough to show up in a small cluster. They usually go away on their own and they aren't contagious, so unlike cold sores and fever blisters, no one can catch a canker sore from kissing you or sharing your drink. But, *man*, are they annoying! Baking soda can help neutralize acids that irritate sores and it kills lingering bacteria in your mouth to help heal your sore quickly. For a cure, try this:

For 1 use

1 teaspoon baking soda

½ cup warm water

1. Combine baking soda and water in a glass. Stir to dissolve.

2. Swish the mixture around in your mouth for several seconds.

3. Spit out the mixture; do not swallow. Repeat once daily, until you experience complete relief.

FOOT ODOR ELIMINATOR

Whether it's your friend, your spouse, or some unfortunate soul on an airplane, we've all been around someone who could knock you over with the smell of their hooves. Stinky feet—bromhidrosis—can happen to anyone, but pregnant women (the injustice!), people who are on their feet all day, anyone who is under a lot of stress, and those with a medical condition called hyperhidrosis, which causes excessive sweating, are especially prone to the condition, which is essentially caused by perspiration. When feet sweat or get wet, bacteria build up and cause odor. The best solution? Keep your little piggies as dry as possible. Thoroughly towel them off after you bathe and use this remedy to keep them smelling fresh.

For 1 use

1 quart warm water
1 tablespoon baking soda

1. In a large bowl or small plastic tub, combine warm water and baking soda.

2. Soak feet for 15 to 20 minutes each night for about one week, or as needed to eliminate odor.

BUG BITE SOOTHER

There's a long list of things I love about summer: sunshine, flip flops, swimming pools, ripe tomatoes, cold beer, fireflies, and backyard barbecues, to name but a few. What's not to love? Well, itchy bug bites can be a real killjoy on a great summer day. Mosquitoes, gnats, biting flies, and other buzzing bugs have a way of really violating your personal space when the weather heats up. Try as we may to repel them, bites from these pesky party crashers are a fact of summertime living. The next time you get a bite, treat it with baking soda to help the itching and swelling subside fast.

For 1 use

1 teaspoon baking soda
A few drops of water or witch hazel

1. Combine baking soda with enough water or witch hazel to make a paste.

2. Spread it on the affected area.

3. Allow paste to remain on skin for 10 to 30 minutes. Rinse with cool water.

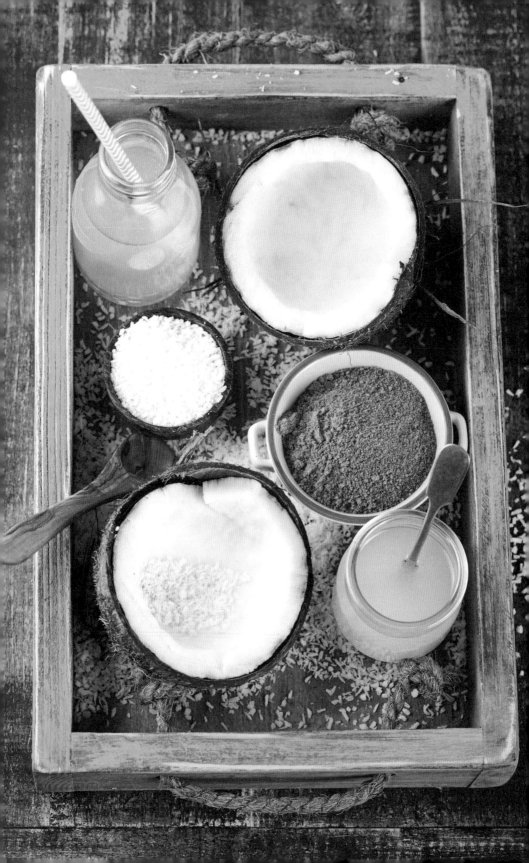

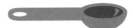

BEAUTY WITH
BAKING SODA

TEETH WHITENER

On a recent visit to our local farmers' market, I was about to buy some locally sourced, artisanal, shade-grown, fair-trade, biodynamic, organic, humanely raised, wild, foraged something-or-other when I heard my husband chuckle. As I looked up at him, he nodded toward a woman walking past us. She was wearing a T-shirt that said "Coffee Until Cocktails." Oh yeah. We know that one! The Mr. and I start every day with coffee and clock out in the evening with a cocktail. I do think about stained teeth in the midst of all that coffee, wine, and sugar. But it's not like we're going to kick the coffee habit or start drinking wine through a straw—I mean, *that* would be insane! Mercifully, we don't have to, because making home-made teeth-whitening paste is a fun and safe way to brighten our smiles!

Makes 3 tablespoons

2 tablespoons hydrogen peroxide
1 tablespoon baking soda

1. Combine hydrogen peroxide and baking soda. Stir into a paste.

2. Brush teeth thoroughly with paste.

3. Leave the paste on your teeth for about a minute, then completely rinse your mouth so that no hydrogen peroxide or baking soda remains.

Note: Limit use of the whitening paste to two or three times a week. Excessive use of baking soda can have the opposite effect of cleaning, breaking down tooth enamel over time and causing sensitivity in your teeth. Make sure you maintain your regular oral care regimen.

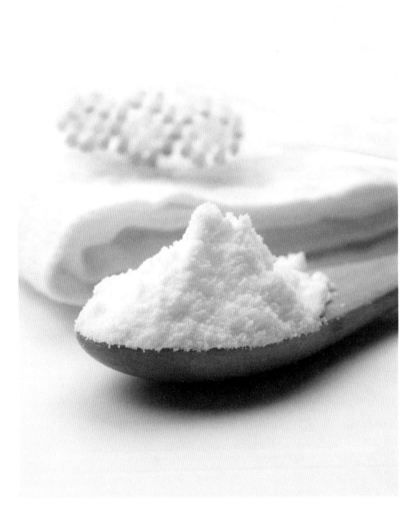

BREATH FRESHENER

It's morning. You've brushed your teeth, used your floss—now for a good, intense swish of breath-freshening mouthwash. Ahhhh. Wait—ow! There's that burn! Yep, most commercial mouthwash—in addition to a cool, minty flavor—contains between 21 and 26 percent alcohol, which not only causes a burning sensation when you use it, but may also have a drying effect on the mouth. Bad breath is caused by excess bacteria giving off excess gas in your mouth. A dry mouth can make bad breath worse, because it encourages the build-up of said bacteria. Baking soda–based mouthwash, on the other hand, neutralizes mouth odors, rather than just covering them up with mint flavoring. Due to its alkaline pH, baking soda balances against acids produced by bacteria and acidic drinks such as sodas and coffee. With this homemade mouthwash, you get a truly clean, fresh smelling mouth without any weird after smell or alcohol burn. This breath freshener works wonders—and it tastes good!

For about 15 uses

2 teaspoons baking soda

10 drops liquid stevia (optional)

10 drops peppermint essential oil

5 drops lemon essential oil

2 cups distilled or purified water

1. Combine all ingredients in a glass jar or bottle.

2. Close the lid tightly and shake the ingredients together for about 30 to 60 seconds. Store in a cool, dark place.

3. To use: Gently shake the bottle and pour a small amount (about an ounce) of mouthwash into a cup, swish it around your mouth for about 30 seconds, then spit. Ahhhhh!

Tip: Did you know that you can use baking soda to turbo-boost your favorite toothpaste? To freshen your mouth and whiten your teeth with ease, squeeze toothpaste onto a wet toothbrush, sprinkle baking soda on top, and scrub away!

HOMEMADE DEODORANT

From workouts to nerves to plain old hot weather, we all need a little *deo* for the *B.O.* every once in a while—the problem lies in all those potentially hazardous chemicals that are in pretty much every stick of deodorant at the drugstore, especially the antiperspirant kind. Maybe it's just the way my brain is hard-wired to the kitchen, but using natural ingredients to nourish my body from the outside as well as the inside just kind of *makes sense.* So I created a recipe for deodorant that does the job without scary chemicals such as aluminum, parabens, phthalates, and other harsh ingredients. You probably have most of what you need to make deodorant in your pantry right now!

Makes about 1½ cups

¼ cup baking soda

¾ cup cornstarch or arrowroot powder

4 to 6 tablespoons melted coconut oil

10 to 15 drops essential oil (optional, but a nice addition— try geranium, lime, rose, or lavender)

1. In a small bowl, combine baking soda and cornstarch or arrowroot.

2. Add 4 tablespoons of melted coconut oil and 10 drops of essential oils and mix with a fork. Continue adding coconut oil and essential oils until the deodorant reaches your desired consistency and fragrance.

3. Store mixture in a jar with a tight-fitting lid.

4. To use, apply a small amount to underarms with your fingertips as needed.

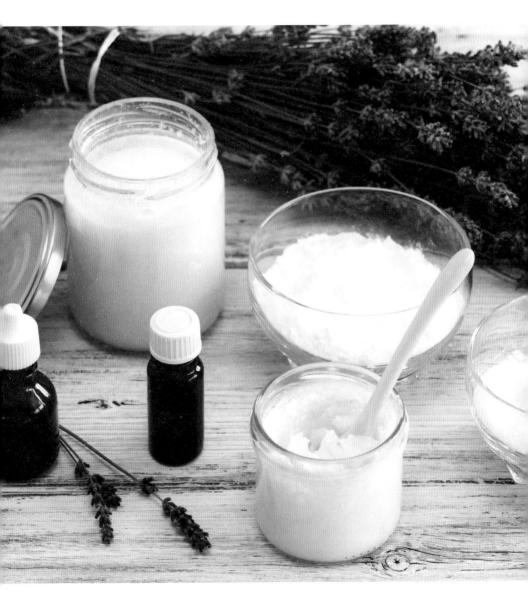

HAIR CARE AU NATURAL

It's no newsflash that using something natural such as baking soda on your hair is greener and healthier than piling on chemical-laden drugstore products, but you may be surprised to know that baking soda actually works like a dream. As in, your hair is going to look not just good, but better than it did before you started using it. I'm all for reducing one's exposure to potentially harmful chemicals, but this mama can't walk around with hair looking like a troll doll's, so I was super-psyched to discover that something as simple as baking soda gave me such great (non-insane looking) results. Here are a few ways to incorporate this ace-in-the-hole in to your hair-care routine.

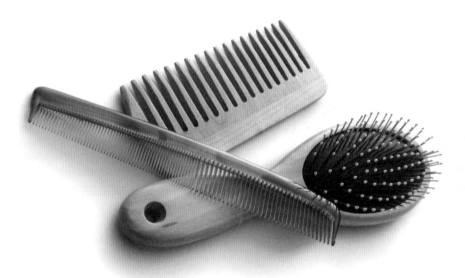

Dry Shampoo

For those days when you've hit the snooze button one time too many and don't have time to wash your hair or when you want to get a little more mileage out of a fabulous blowout:

For 3 to 4 uses

½ cup cornstarch (or unsweetened cocoa powder for dark hair)

2 tablespoons baking soda

A few drops essential oil of your choice (optional)

1. Combine cornstarch or cocoa powder (or a combination of the two), baking soda, and essential oils, if using, in a small glass jar, ideally with a shaker top. (I like to reuse old spice jars.)

2. To use the dry shampoo, sprinkle a small amount on your hair just at the scalp area. Allow the powder to absorb the dirt and oils for a minute or two, then flip your hair upside down, use your fingers to blend the powder, shake out your roots, and allow the dry shampoo to move toward your ends. Give your hair a quick brush, then hit the road.

Continued

Anti-Dandruff Treatment

Skip the shampoo and go right to rinsing after using this treatment. You may find that your hair feels a bit dry at first, but after a few weeks, your scalp's natural oil production will reset itself, leaving your hair softer and free of flakes.

For 1 use

¼ cup rosewater or tap water
¼ cup baking soda

1. Mix rosewater or water and baking soda to make a paste.

2. Apply paste to your scalp and gently massage for 2 to 3 minutes.

3. Rinse thoroughly with cool water.

Après-Swim Shampoo

When you and your hair have diametrically opposed opinions about whether spending time in the pool is a good thing, this simple treatment makes peace after sun and chlorine exposure.

For 1 use

1 tablespoon baking soda
1 cup water

1. Combine baking soda and water.

2. Apply mixture directly to hair. (If your hair feels slimy while you're washing it with the solution, it's working!)

3. Rinse the mixture with clean water, then follow with your normal hair-care routine.

Brush and Comb Cleaner

Brushing or combing clean hair with a hairbrush that's been accumulating dirt, germs, and product gunk for who-knows-how-long is . . . well, it's pretty gross, isn't it? For great-looking hair and longer-lasting brushes and combs, clean regularly.

For 1 use

A sink full of warm water
1 to 2 teaspoons baking soda

1. Rake through the bristles of your hairbrush using a comb or your fingers to remove as much of the old hair trapped in the bristles as possible.

2. Fill a sink up with warm water and add baking soda. Soak brushes and combs in the baking soda solution for 20 to 30 minutes.

3. Rinse well with warm/hot water.

4. Allow brushes and combs to dry thoroughly.

HOMEMADE FACIAL SCRUB

Is it just me or is a scrub everyone's favorite facial product? A good scrub brightens everything right up by rubbing away icky dead skin cells and cleaning out your pores—so satisfying! My former-favorite scrub was a name-brand product that had little microbeads suspended in glistening gel, but because it turns out that those tiny plastic particles are incredibly harmful to the environment and, ultimately, not so great for your skin, I had to find a new way to exfoliate. Lo and behold, the road to perfectly polished skin is paved with baking soda! Simple, cheap, and all natural—here's how.

For 1 to 2 uses

1 tablespoon baking soda
1 tablespoon honey

Combine equal parts baking soda and honey in the palm of your hand. Massage into clean, damp skin in circular motions. Rinse with water.

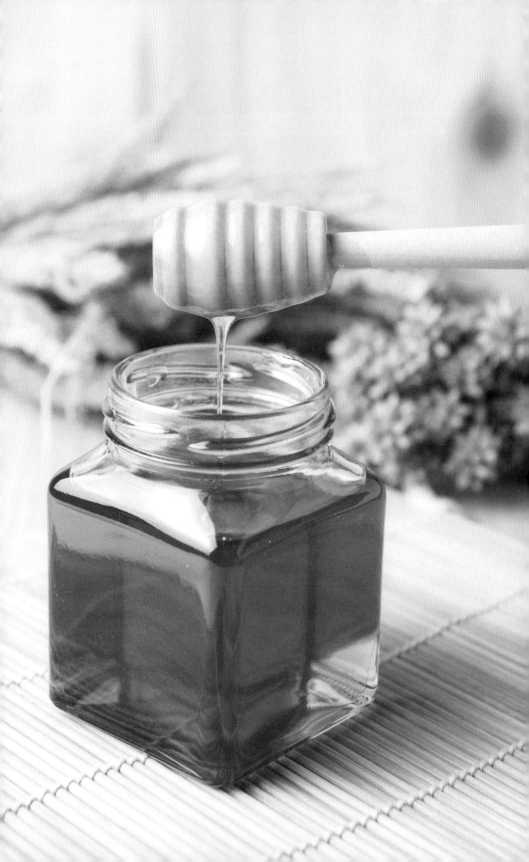

SKIN BRIGHTENER

When I was in my twenties, I could burn the candle at both ends, exist on not-quite-enough sleep, and still look fresh—kinda effortlessly. Not long ago, I had the startling realization that nowadays when I'm tired from too much work or too much . . . life, I *look* it. I mean, REALLY. In a panic, I started to stockpile fake-it-till-you-make-it products in an attempt to achieve a more pulled-together, seemingly rested appearance (friends, do not underestimate the power of an illuminating highlighter). I also heard about an all-natural skin brightener that works like an energy drink for the skin and costs a whole lot less than other brightening products I'd bought at fancy cosmetic counters. I tried it and—whoa—definitely looked fresher! Like I'd slept *at least* 7 hours. Try it.

For 1 use

1 tablespoon baking soda

1 teaspoon lemon juice (more or less, to achieve a medium-thin paste)

A few drops of warm water

1. In a small bowl, combine baking soda with lemon juice and enough water to achieve a medium-thin paste.

2. Smooth the mixture onto your face and leave it for 5 to 10 minutes, or until it dries completely.

3. Rinse thoroughly and pat dry to reveal brighter skin. Use no more than once or twice weekly.

DIY ACNE MASK

Funny, isn't it, how you can more or less count on a break-out sneaking up on you just before a big event such as a job interview or your best friend's wedding? More than once, I've found myself deep in panic mode after catching my reflection in an airplane bathroom mirror, finding a surprise zit staring back at me, and knowing I hadn't packed any sort of blemish buster in my toiletry bag. If you find yourself face to face with skin problems—either a one-off pimple or more regular skin freakouts—there's no need to slather on an over-the-counter zit zapper, which can be full of nasty, skin-irritating chemicals anyway. Simply whip up this simple, natural, baking soda mask and get glowing, gorgeous skin overnight!

Makes 1 mask

1 teaspoon baking soda

1 tablespoon honey

½ teaspoon cinnamon

1. Cleanse your face thoroughly.

2. Combine baking soda, honey, and cinnamon together in a small bowl.

3. Apply mixture to your face in one even coat.

4. Leave on for 15 to 20 minutes.

5. Rinse thoroughly with warm water and follow with soothing face lotion.

BLACKHEAD REMOVER

Here's a fun dermatologic fact: A blackhead is a pimple that doesn't have any skin over it. Weird, right? It's just a zit at the skin's surface instead of underneath, like a whitehead. Because there's nothing covering the gunk in the pore, and it's exposed to the air, the stuff oxidizes and turns dark, almost black in color. Hence the name: *black*head. If you have a tendency to get blackheads, I have good and bad news for you. The bad news is that it probably means you have large pores and oily skin, which takes a bit of work to keep under control. The good news is that you probably won't wrinkle as quickly as you age, because your skin's oils keep it moister and smoother. So when you're 60, you'll probably look 40. Think of that! Meanwhile, you're going to want to deal with those pesky little dark spots, which are probably taking up real estate on your nose and in your T-zone. A little baking soda goes a long way toward banishing blackheads. Its tiny, fine granules work to exfoliate and remove anything clogging your pores, leaving you with smooth, blackhead-free skin.

For 1 use

1 to 2 tablespoons water
1 tablespoon baking soda

1. Mix water with baking soda to form a thick but spreadable paste.

2. Using a gentle, circular motion, massage the paste into your skin for a minute or two.

3. Rinse thoroughly with cool water, pat your face dry, then moisturize with a gentle lotion.

Note: To effectively deal with blackheads, all you need to do is clean out your pores and those suckers will be ejected from your face. There's no need to pinch, squish, and squeeze, which can lead to scarring and infection. If you just have to pop something, go get yourself a roll of bubble wrap!

SHAVING BUTTER

What do Duane "The Rock" Johnson, Patrick Stewart, post-'90s Bruce Willis, and my husband all have in common? They're debonair gentlemen who have embraced their clean-domed selves and emerged all the better for it. I can't speak for the majority of that list, but I do know that my husband has some pretty strong opinions when it comes to shaving cream. As well he should! The guy regularly shaves everything above the neck (minus eyebrows) each time he picks up a razor, so he knows a thing or two about how to get the job done. His shaving cream must-have list includes protection from nicks and cuts, moisturizing, and a nice scent. Most canned drugstore shaving creams are loaded with chemicals that can dry out the skin. On the other hand, the "natural" shaving soaps and creams he's tried and liked tend to come with a hefty price tag. I discovered, however, another option, which is to make a super-moisturizing shaving cream at home. It isn't difficult and doing so offers the freedom to choose the ingredients you like and avoid those you don't. This recipe makes a pretty healthy quantity. My husband, who only shaves a few times a week, keeps a few shaves' worth in a covered container in the bathroom, then refills from the stash in the refrigerator when he runs out.

Makes about 1 cup

¼ cup olive, almond, or coconut oil

2 to 3 tablespoons shea or cocoa butter

¼ cup aloe gel or honey

1 tablespoon cornstarch

¼ cup liquid castille soap

10 to 15 drops essential oil (see tips)

2 teaspoons baking soda

1. Place all the ingredients except the essential oils and baking soda in a small saucepan. Melt over low heat, stirring occasionally until it liquefies, then remove the pan from heat.

2. Add 10 to 15 drops of essential oil. Stir well to combine.

3. Pour the mixture into a mixing bowl, cover, and refrigerate for an hour or two, until thoroughly chilled. The mixture will solidify slightly.

4. Remove from refrigerator, add baking soda and, using an electric mixer or a whisk, beat the mixture until it becomes light and fluffy.

5. Transfer shaving cream to a jar or another container with a tight-fitting lid. Store it in a cool, dark place until you're ready to use it.

Tips: Clove, cedarwood, sage, and bergamot essential oils work nicely to acheive a "masculine" scent, but use any oils you like. If you like a foamier shaving cream, try using an old-school shaving brush to achieve a nice lather.

HAND AND CUTICLE TREATMENT

Because I use my hands a lot—for cooking, obviously, but also for lots of gardening and DIY projects around the house—my fingers end up taking a bit of a beating. Uneven nails, chipped polish, ragged cuticles, and dry hands aren't really that big a deal in the big scheme of things, but I *am* a professional after all and people in my cooking classes, for example, don't need to look at my hands and think "What's going on here? Did she just break out of prison? Did she spend all night digging ditches?" So I rely on a few baking-soda-centric hand and nail treatments to keep it all tidy between visits to the nail salon.

Nail Smoother

Use this smoother to banish nicks and smooth ridges on your nail surface.

For 1 use

1 tablespoon baking soda
1 teaspoon water

1. Combine baking soda and water to create a paste.

2. Rub gently in circular motions over fingernails to smooth the nail surface.

3. Rinse clean with warm water, file, and apply polish as usual.

Cuticle Exfoliator

Instead of cutting cuticles, scrub them to remove dead skin cells and to smooth cracked cuticles.

For 1 use

2 teaspoons baking soda
2 teaspoons water

1. Using a wooden cuticle stick or a terry cloth towel, gently push back cuticles.

2. Combine baking soda and water to create a paste.

3. Gently run paste on fingers in a circular motion, concentrating on the area surrounding the nail bed.

4. Rinse clean with warm water, file, and apply polish as usual.

SMOOTHING, SOOTHING, AND SOFTENING FOOT TREATMENT

I never really noticed how dry and rough my feet could be until I met my husband. Not because he'd commented on my less-than-silky feet—he's too nice a guy for that—but because I'd noticed how freakishly soft and smooth his were in comparison to mine. (And, by the way, he comes by it 100 percent naturally. I thought *maybe* he had some kind of awesome secret treatment he was hiding, but, nope, he's just a man who happens to have really soft feet. Seriously, folks, like a baby's.) Even though I was a regular in the pedicure chair, I guess between exercise, high heels, sandals, and probably some straight-up neglect, I was sporting some rough, cracked, funky feet. Clearly, I needed to step up my foot-care game. I stumbled upon an emergency rescue plan, compliments of baking soda, and was able to get my feet back into fighting shape in no time. Use this treatment a few times a week and enjoy softer, smoother, happier feet.

For 1 use

2 to 3 tablespoons baking soda, plus more for scrubbing

A few drops of essential oil (optional)

Clean warm water (enough to fill a small tub or foot bath)

1. Combine baking soda and essential oils (if using) with enough warm water to fill a small tub or foot bath.

2. Immerse your feet and allow them to soak for 15 to 20 minutes.

3. Next, scrub trouble spots, such as the heels and balls of the feet, with a mixture of baking soda and enough water to form a paste.

4. Rinse with clean water, then pat dry.

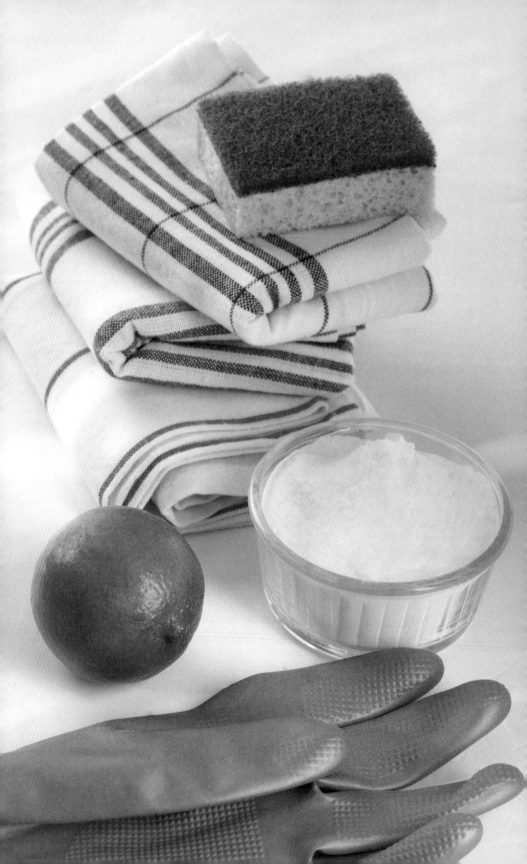

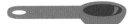

CLEANING WITH
BAKING SODA

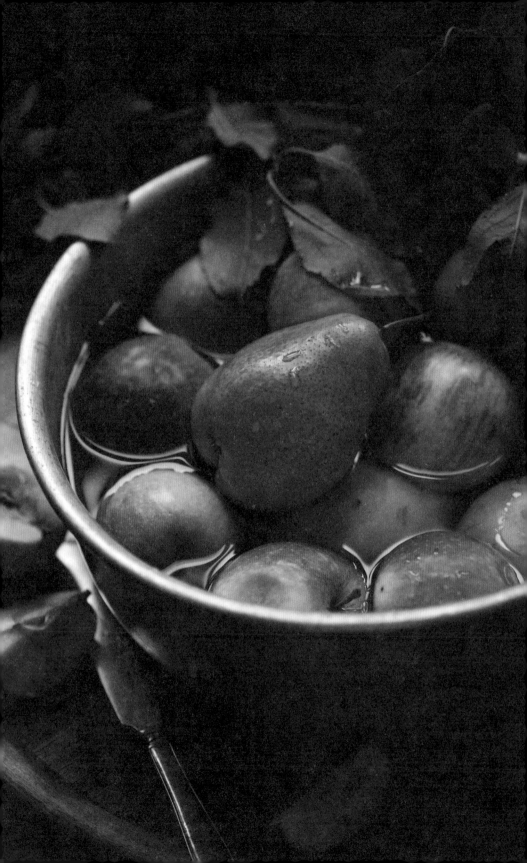

FRUIT AND VEGETABLE WASH

I know it seems tedious, but even if you stick to buying organic, it's important to wash your produce before you eat it to get rid of icky germs, bugs, waxes, pesticide residue, and any other slimy, grimy surprises that may be lurking in your farm-fresh treasures. Sure, plain old water works to remove surface dirt and sand, but a fruit and vegetable wash can help you get the job of cleaning done more thoroughly, plus it allows you to use less water in the process—bonus! Making your own produce wash at home is quick and easy, so no need to buy one of those pricey commercial fruit and vegetable sprays. Simply mix, spray, and let the ingredients shine.

Makes 2 cups

1 cup water

1 cup distilled white vinegar

1 tablespoon baking soda

20 drops grapefruit seed extract (available at most health food stores, or substitute ¼ teaspoon lemon juice)

1. Combine all ingredients in a large container.

2. Transfer to a spray bottle, ideally the kind with a pump, which allows you to apply a thin, even mist on produce.

3. Spray mixture on produce and allow to sit 5 to 10 minutes. Rinse thoroughly with cool water.

CUTTING BOARD CLEANER

Allow me to assume that if you are reading this page, then you are like most people. Meaning, you are a person who owns at least one cutting board. If your cutting board is made of plastic, skip to the next page to read why you should consider using a wooden one; meanwhile go ahead and toss your plastic board in the dishwasher, because that's the easiest way to clean it. Boom. Done. And by the way, please, please, pleeeeeease do not use a glass, metal, or marble cutting board. Why? First of all: the sound of a knife on glass. Eeeeeeek. But also, those surfaces are way too hard on your knife blade. We're talking about a one-way ticket to Dullsville. If, however, you are the lucky owner of a wooden cutting board, then we need to chat about the complicated relationship you're involved in. You see, to keep a wooden board in good working order, you've got to give it a little extra love and attention. To clean and sanitize it, you can't just chuck it into the dishwasher. That'll crack and warp your board. But you can easily keep your board beautiful and clean—just follow these easy steps.

For 1 use

¼ to ½ cup kosher salt

1 to 2 tablespoons lemon juice

¼ to ½ cup baking soda

1 to 2 tablespoons water

Mineral oil or another food-grade oil that isn't prone to rancidity

WHY WOOD WINS

For everyday use, a wooden cutting board is the friendliest kind of cutting board you'll find. Not only is it prettier and gentler on your knife blade than other materials, but wood is actually the safest material as far as food-borne bacteria goes. It turns out, plastic cutting boards retain bacteria in the nicks and scars left behind by your knife blade—even after scrubbing and washing in the dishwasher. Sure, wood retains food-borne bacteria, too, even after hand washing with soapy hot water, but the difference is that it *absorbs* the bacteria inside and holds it there, where it simply can't multiply and eventually dies. Studies have found that, even when a cootie-ridden wooden cutting board is sliced open with a sharp knife, the bacteria don't come out. Wood (somehow) kills them! Best. Cutting. Board. Ever.

To keep your board clean on a daily basis:

1. In the center of your board, pour ¼ to ½ cup of kosher salt, depending on the size—bigger boards need more salt. Add enough lemon juice to make a paste.

2. Using a sponge or cloth, scour the board thoroughly, then rinse with clean water.

Once a week:

1. Pour between ¼ and ½ cup of baking soda (again depending on the cutting board's size) onto your still-damp cutting board. Add enough water to make a paste.

2. Using a sponge or cloth, scour the board thoroughly. You may find that odors are released from the board during this step. If it stinks, you're doing good work!

Continued

3. Rinse thoroughly with clean water and dry with cloth or paper towels. Allow to air dry completely.

Every couple of weeks or whenever your board starts to look dry or otherwise unhappy:

1. Using a clean, soft cloth or paper towel, apply the mineral oil in an even layer over the wood. Allow the oil to soak in for at least a few hours, ideally overnight.

2. Remove the excess oil by rubbing it with a clean, dry cloth or paper towel.

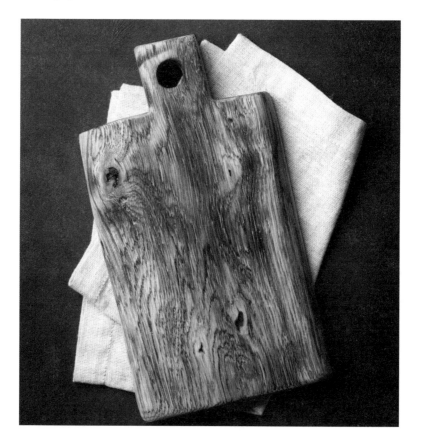

DIY DISHWASHING POWDER

This "recipe" emerged as a result of laziness and desperation on the part of yours truly. I was rushing around one afternoon, getting things ready for dinner guests, when I realized that I had a dishwasher full of dirty dishes and no dishwashing detergent. Sure, I *could* have run out to the store to replenish the supply, and I suppose I could have washed all of the dishes by hand (hahahaha) but instead I decided to check in with my dear friend The Internet to see if I could substitute something such as laundry soap (you can't) or my beloved baking soda (bingo!) to get them clean in a pinch. All it takes is a few drops of liquid dish soap and some baking soda to get your dishes squeaky clean.

For 1 use

2 drops liquid dish soap (That's it! Any more and you'll have suds everywhere!)

2 tablespoons baking soda

1. Squeeze liquid dish soap into the soap compartment of your dishwasher.

2. Add baking soda to the compartment or toss onto the floor of the machine.

3. Run the dishwasher as you would normally.

4. Never worry about running out of dishwasher soap again!

ALL-PURPOSE KITCHEN CLEANER

No doubt about it, cooking—and eating—is messy business. From sticky countertops to splattered floors and everything in between, you need a dependable product to clean up dirt, grease, crumbs, and spills. With a handful of supplies, you can quickly and easily make your own all-natural kitchen cleaner, which is both good for your wallet and your health. Plus, the recipe below is as pure and simple as baking soda, vinegar, and water, so look at you being all green! Nice one.

Makes 2 cups

1 teaspoon baking soda
½ teaspoon liquid dish soap
2 tablespoons distilled white vinegar
Warm water
Essential oil (optional)

1. Combine baking soda, dish soap, and vinegar in a 16-ounce spray bottle.

2. Stir or shake vigorously, then allow mixture to settle for a minute or two.

3. Fill the bottle with warm water and a few drops of essential oil, if desired. Shake again, then get to cleaning!

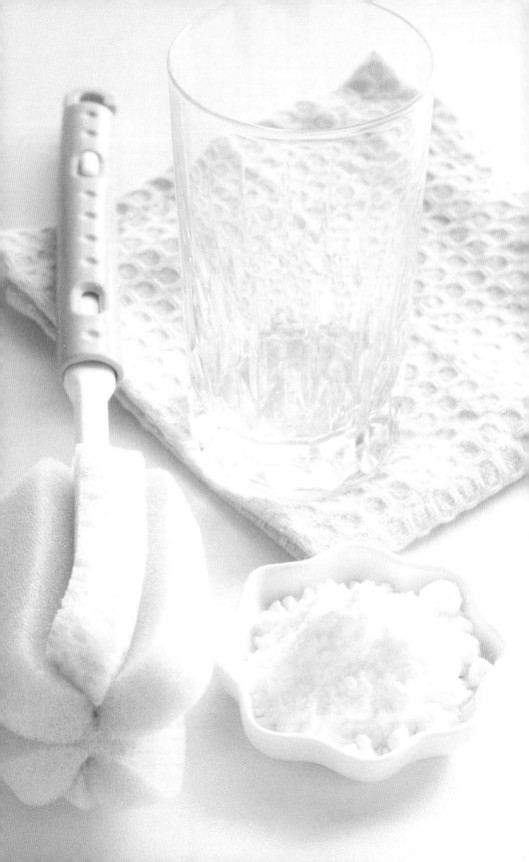

BATHROOM CLEANERS

Confession: I don't always practice what I preach. I love the idea of simple, natural cleaning products, especially ones I can make myself, and have used them in most rooms of my house for some time. But never in the bathroom. The bathroom is a different story entirely. The bathroom is like another universe, where "dirty" means something else. The bathroom is, well . . . it's gross! So, for a very long time, I was addicted to chemical-laden cleaning products that could transform a nasty, germ-ridden bathroom into a disinfected, sparkling, lemon-scented retreat. I knew that what I was using probably wasn't safe for my family or the environment, but I'm ashamed to admit that I didn't care, because I wanted it Clean with a capital C. Then we moved into a house with extremely hard water that left ugly, impossible-to-remove stains on our beautiful glass shower door. I scrubbed the heck out of that door and tried tons of products, one of which you can learn all about from a late-night infomercial. Nothing worked. Nothing, that is, except for baking soda, which worked like a charm on the first try. From that moment I was sold on its power to clean absolutely ANY-THING, including the bathroom. From the toilet to the shower curtain, use these tips to get your bathroom clean—no 1-800 number required.

Toilet Cleaner

For 1 use

1 cup baking soda
Distilled white vinegar

1. Sprinkle the toilet with 1 cup of baking soda.

2. Let it sit for 30 minutes, then spray or squirt with enough vinegar to moisten.

3. Scrub with a toilet brush, then flush.

Surface and Soap Scum Cleaner

For 1 use

1 cup baking soda
1 cup liquid dish soap

1. Wipe down tubs and sinks with a damp sponge or cloth.

2. Combine baking soda and liquid dish soap to make a paste.

3. Scrub tub and sink surfaces thoroughly, then rinse clean with water.

Continued

Shower Door Cleaner

For 1 use

Sprinkle a little baking soda on a damp sponge and wipe down the glass. Rinse well and dry. For a really impressive finish, use a squeegee to remove lint and streaks.

Marble and Stone Surface Cleaner

For 1 use

½ cup baking soda
¼ cup water

Coat stains with a thick paste made from 2 parts baking soda to 1 part water. Give the mixture 24 to 48 hours to draw out the stains, then rinse and dry the surface thoroughly.

Grout Cleaner

For 1 use

½ cup baking soda
½ cup water

Make a thin paste with equal parts baking soda and water. Using an old toothbrush, gently scrub the grout. If you think you're dealing with mold or a fungus, knock it out with a thicker mixture of three parts baking soda to one part bleach (it's OK every once in a while!). Rinse either mixture with plenty of water and dry thoroughly.

Shower Curtain Cleaner

For 1 use

½ cup baking soda

Regular laundry detergent

½ cup distilled white vinegar (optional)

1. Shower curtains (both cloth and vinyl) can be machine-washed with baking soda. Add ½ cup baking soda along with your regular detergent and set the machine to the gentle cycle. (Tossing in a few towels will keep a vinyl curtain from sticking to itself and clumping.)

2. To really disinfect, pour in ½ cup vinegar during the rinse cycle.

3. Let a vinyl curtain air-dry (it will melt in the dryer—and even I'm not sure how much baking soda it would take to clean up that mess!)

AIR FRESHENER

I love a fragranced room. Sicilian tangerine-scented candles, cucumber and lotus flower–infused sticks, English pear and freesia room spray . . . I have dropped some bank in the name of home fragrance. Although, as much as I love using air fresheners—and let's be clear: I LOVE them—I've come to the profound realization that many of my beloved scents (yes, even you, Japanese Black Currant) simply mask odors instead of actually eradicating them. When I have to contend with a considerable stench—especially, of the kitcheny or bathroomy variety—I use an air freshener made with baking soda, which actually neutralizes bad smells (see: your fridge). It's incredibly easy to put together and can even be customized to appeal to those of us who need a little orange blossom and cedar leaf in our lives. This room freshener continually emits a light scent while the baking soda works to absorb any unwanted odors. When you need more fragrance, just give it a little shake!

Makes 1 air freshener

½ cup baking soda

15 to 25 drops essential oil(s) of your choice

A small jar with a perforated lid, such as a clean, empty parmesan shaker or a ½-pint mason jar with a pin-pricked piece of card stock in place of the lid—secure it with the mason jar ring

1. Combine baking soda essential oil(s) in the prepared jar. With your hand over the lid's holes, shake well to evenly distribute the oils.

2. Decorate, if you like.

3. Place your air freshener jar anywhere you want to control odors, such as bathrooms, trash areas, closets, etc.

4. Shake your air freshener jar frequently to keep the scent activated. If you notice that the fragrance starts to fade, simply add 4 to 5 drops of additional essential oil to jar.

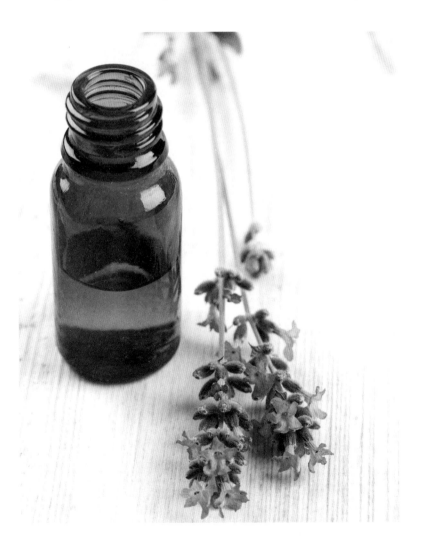

SILVER POLISH

Not long ago, my parents decided to downsize from a house to an apartment. To get ready, a considerable amount of organizing and consolidating needed to take place, so I made a trip to help with The Great Purge. One afternoon, my mom and I spent time on a closet that housed all sorts of table linens, serving pieces, and an incredible amount of silver, including a tea set, large platters, tiny salt bowls, flatware for 12, a gravy boat, and quite a few things I couldn't identify, all of which she kept meticulously wrapped in these special anti-tarnish cloths. (Because, evidently, light and air are enemies to silver.) With the exception of a few platters, my mom explained that she wouldn't have space to store most of the silver in their new place—plus she was no longer interested in "all that upkeep"—but did I want any of it? *Did* I want any of it?! I tried to be forward-thinking and consider all the occasions down the road when it would be nice to present a turkey on my great aunt's (ginormous) silver platter or to serve spiced nuts at a party in my grandmother's little silver bowls, but "all that upkeep" kept reverberating in my head. I imagined myself wearing a frilly apron, curlers in my hair, sweat on my brow, elbow deep in pasty, smelly silver polish. I can't even find time to iron! In the end, I agreed to take a few very simple serving pieces, which do sometimes reside in the darkness of their anti-tarnish cloaks, because I am still a wee bit intimidated by "all that upkeep." However, I'm happy to report that when I do use the stuff, I have a lightning fast, almost magic way to get that silver spiffed up and event ready.

Continued

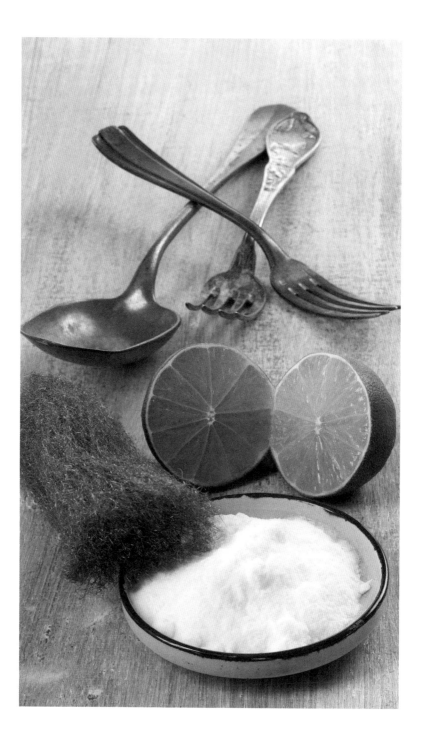

For 1 use

Mild dish soap

Aluminum foil

2 cups boiling water

2 tablespoons baking soda

1 teaspoon salt

1. Hand wash items to be cleaned in warm, soapy water.

2. Place silver pieces in an aluminum foil-lined pan, such as a glass baking dish.

3. In a pitcher or bowl, combine 1 quart boiling water with baking soda and salt. Pour the mixture over the silver and allow it to sit for 30 seconds to 5 minutes as the solution works to remove any tarnish from the silver.

4. Remove silver from pan, rinse with clean water, and dry with a clean, soft cloth.

RUST ELIMINATOR

I always imagined that cleaning rust was a complicated endeavor that involved the use of a metal brush and some sort of thick paste that you'd apply with steel wool while wearing heavy gloves. Just the idea of it caused me to feel annoyed and exhausted. Which is why, when I finally came to terms with the fact that I had to do something about the rusted-out corners of my favorite sheet pan (or else say goodbye), I became instantly cranky and may or may not have whined loudly, "I don't wanna!" To save that pan, I needed a shortcut, because I would NOT, under any circumstances, be wielding a metal brush. I'd used baking soda and lemon juice plenty of times to clean other kinds of grime off metal, so I figured it was worth a try on the rusty pan. I made a paste, slapped it on, then left it there while I went about my business for an hour and when I returned . . . success! The rust wiped off easily and completely. Slacker way wins!

For 1 use

⅓ cup baking soda

3 tablespoons lemon juice (or lime juice if you want to imagine you're drinking a margarita instead of doing housework)

1. Combine baking soda and lemon or lime juice to make a paste.

2. Apply to rusted surfaces and allow to sit for 30 to 60 minutes.

3. Using a damp sponge or rag, scrub lightly to remove rust, then rinse thoroughly with plain water.

ECO-FRIENDLY PEST CONTROL

Maybe it's all those summers I spent in the woods at camp when I was a kid, but I am not particularly squeamish about bugs when I'm outside (annoyed, perhaps, by the biting and stinging sorts, but not squeamish). I appreciate creatures such as garden worms, ladybugs, and spiders for their unique and important contributions to our ecosystem. *Inside* my house, however, I am not so hospitable. To keep out uninvited guests, such as ants and roaches, I use a simple yet surprisingly effective solution of sugar and baking soda. The sugar attracts the insect and the baking soda kills it. To protect your home from the creepy crawlies, try this earth-friendly, nontoxic solution.

Makes 2 bait dishes

1 tablespoon sugar (for ants, use powdered sugar)
1 tablespoon baking soda

1. Combine sugar and baking soda.

2. Add a tablespoon or so into a small dish or container (the lid from an old jar works well).

3. Repeat, placing more small dishes behind appliances, inside of cupboards and pantries, in the garage, and anywhere you might suspect roaches to live and breed.

4. When you see dead roaches around the bait, replenish the dish. (And get rid of the dead roaches!)

Note: The process may take weeks before you see the benefit. Since the sugar and baking soda are not pesticides, they will not act as quickly as chemicals, but are much safer for your family and pets.

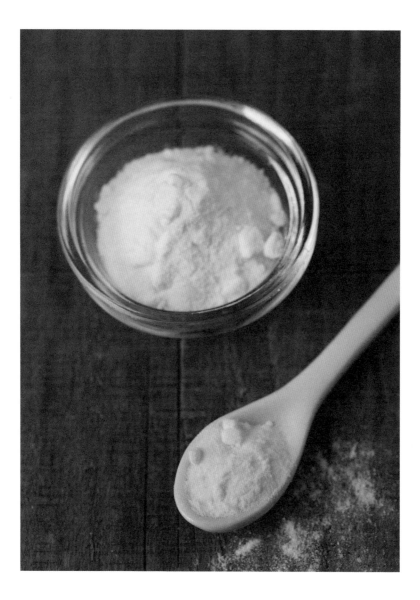

DRAIN DE-CLOGGER

We have a bathroom in our house that gets a lot of traffic. It's used for typical bathroom sink purposes, such as washing one's hands after one has *gone*; brushing one's teeth in the get-out-the-door-fast morning frenzy; setting up a Barbie doll hair salon; conducting experiments in which crayons are wrapped in wads of toilet paper and then submerged in a sink full of soapy water, which, ultimately, gets abandoned for an hour or more—y'know, typical stuff. Needless to say, it tends to drain slowly from time to time, and every few months, when my husband or I notice that water is moving slower than a tortoise, we go at it with baking soda and vinegar. Far cheaper and much safer for your pipes (and the environment), this technique is effective for kitchen and bathroom clogs and is—I do confess—kind of fun!

For 1 use

1 cup baking soda
1 cup distilled white vinegar
Boiling water

1. Remove the drain cover. (Many drain covers thread into the drain, so try unscrewing it by turning it to the left.)

2. Using a cloth or paper towel, dry inside of the sink or tub.

3. Pour baking soda down the drain, followed by the vinegar. The mixture will foam vigorously.

4. Allow baking soda and vinegar to remain for about 5 minutes.

5. Carefully, pour several cups of boiling water down the drain. This should clear it.

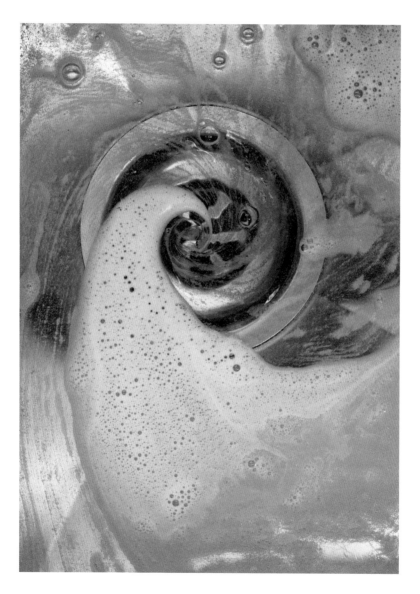

COFFEEPOT CLEANER

If you've got a coffee maker, then chances are you know you should clean it every once in a while. Funny how knowing we should do something and actually doing it are not quite the same. In any case, regular cleaning of your coffee machine is a good thing. But why? Well, for starters it'll help ensure great-tasting coffee. Oily residue, hard-water deposits, and other gunk build up in coffee makers over time. The result: bitter, funky-tasting brew. Plus, regular cleaning will remove hard water spots from the carafe and prevent staining. Also, a good cleaning every now and again will keep the machine in good working order, so you can keep brewing awesome coffee! This simple method works on automatic drip coffee makers as well as pod-style machines.

For 1 use

Warm water
¼ cup baking soda

1. Fill your coffeepot or the reservoir of your pod-style machine with warm water.

2. Add baking soda and stir until dissolved.

3. Pour the baking soda solution into the chamber of your coffee maker and run the machine as you normally would when brewing a pot of coffee. For pod-style machines, close the pod chamber, then run as though you're brewing a cup.

4. When the brew cycle has finished, discard the baking soda water and rinse the carafe or cup thoroughly.

5. Run the brew cycle two more times with clean water, rinsing the carafe or cup thoroughly between cycles.

6. Repeat every 2 to 6 weeks, depending on frequency of use.

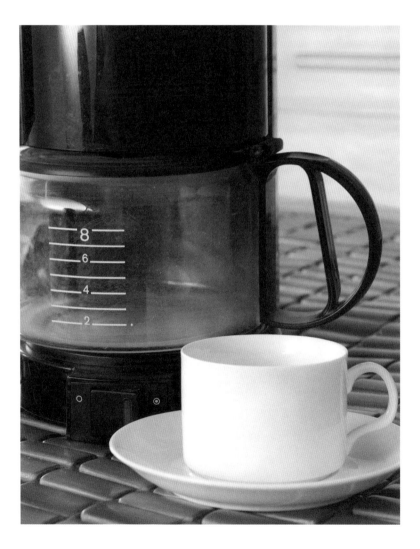

FRIDGE ODOR ELIMINATOR

Storing an opened box of baking soda in your refrigerator and freezer to help eliminate odors is pretty much baking soda 101, isn't it? But what about tough refrigerator odors? The kind of odors that are emitted from office break room refrigerators or fraternity house refrigerators or your very own refrigerator that stinks for no apparent reason, even though you threw out that green, fuzzy pan of mystery leftovers a week ago . . . For those kinds of odors you need to do a little more than just crack open a box of baking soda. Here's how to return even the rankest fridge to fresh-smelling status quo.

For 1 use

½ cup distilled white vinegar
2 gallons warm water
1 cup baking soda
Liquid dish soap

1. Empty the entire contents of your refrigerator. If you have a second fridge, stash perishables there. Otherwise, store them in a freestanding cooler.

2. Remove the shelves, bins, crisper drawers, and any other removable parts and hand-wash them in hot, soapy water with the liquid dish soap.

3. In a clean bucket or tub, combine vinegar with 1 gallon of water and use the solution to wipe the bins and shelves

down; rinse with clean water. Dry thoroughly with cloth or paper towels.

4. Combine baking soda with 1 gallon of water and use the solution to wipe down the inside of the refrigerator. Dry thoroughly with cloth or paper towels.

5. Restock.

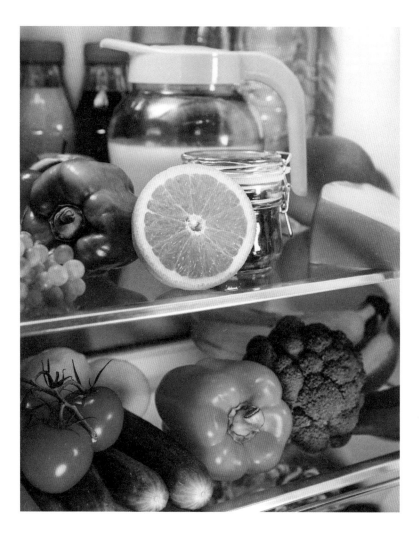

MICROWAVE CLEANER

Keeping the microwave clean isn't always easy (especially if your microwave is mounted above your stove and you are an adult under 5 feet tall and can't actually see all the way into the microwave unless you are standing on a stepping stool). It's a time-consuming task and, let's be honest, if you're using the microwave, you're probably already looking to save time. This quick method takes just 18 minutes, 17 and a half of which are unattended, and results in a splatter-free, spill-free, odor-free microwave.

For 1 use

2 tablespoons baking soda

1 cup water

1. Combine baking soda and water in a microwave-safe container.

2. Microwave the mixture on high for 3 minutes.

3. Leave the container in the microwave with the door closed for 15 minutes.

4. Using oven mitts, carefully remove the container from the microwave.

5. With a damp cloth, wipe out the inside of the microwave and door.

6. Use paper or cloth towels to thoroughly dry the inside of the microwave or allow it to air dry with the door open.

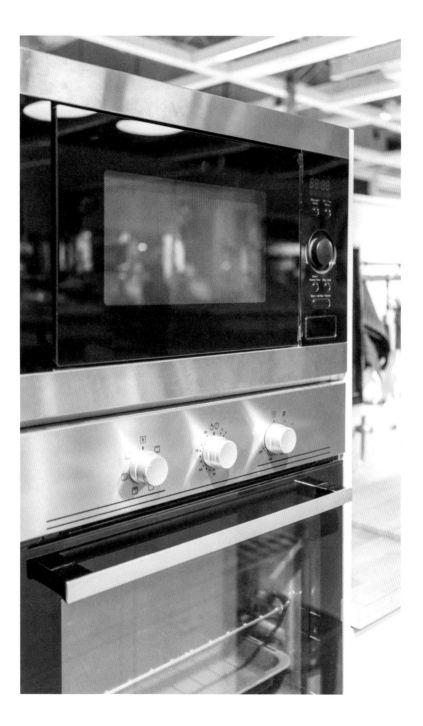

STAINLESS STEEL COOKWARE SALVATION

There's nothing like a new stainless steel saucepan: so shiny, so new, so very good-looking! But stainless steel is more than just a pretty face—stainless steel cookware is a hustler that can go from stovetop to oven with ease, has a surface that browns food beautifully and turns out great pan sauces like a boss. Save for a few instances when I prefer the weight and history of my cast-iron skillet, stainless steel is my go-to choice for everyday use. As much as I love it, I confess that stainless isn't as easy to clean as, say, nonstick. Over time it can end up with unsightly brown spots and that just won't go away with regular dishwashing. Thankfully, no matter how banged up your pots and pans get, there is a super inexpensive and simple way to get them looking new again. It does require a little bit of muscle, but the outcome is totally worth the sweat.

For 1 use

Water

1 to 2 tablespoons baking soda

1. Pour a very small amount of water into the pot to be cleaned, then add baking soda.

2. Mix the water and baking soda together to form a loose paste.

3. Using a sponge, spread the paste all around the pot, including up the sides and on the outside of the pot.

4. Using some muscle and stamina, have at those stains! You may find that you need to add more baking soda and spend a few extra minutes on the stubborn stains.

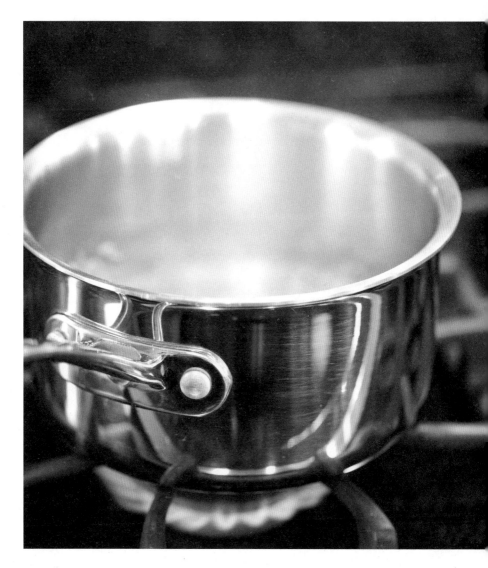

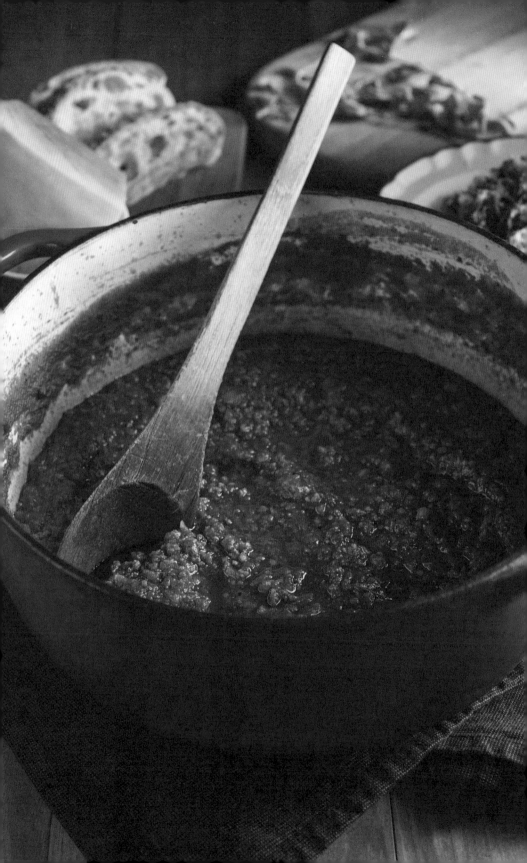

ENAMELED CAST-IRON COOKWARE CLEANER

Of all the cookware I own, I'm most attached to my big, red hulk of a Dutch oven. It was a wedding gift and has turned out some pretty memorable meals in its time. Now guess what happened when a call from the pediatrician, a new rug delivery, and a never-saw-it-coming decision on the part of my kids to finger-paint *each other* coincided with said Dutch oven being left unattended, full of sautéing onions? Bingo: a horrific, black, burnt-on mess. Tragic. Not only was dinner a bust, I worried "Big Red" was a goner. Happily, though, I was able to save the pot with baking soda. I recommend this method not only for burnt-on disasters, but as preventative care for keeping your enameled cookware in tip-top shape. I also recommend storing finger paints on a high shelf. Lesson learned.

For 1 use

1 quart water
2 tablespoons baking soda

1. Pour the water into the pot to be cleaned, and then bring it to a boil over medium heat.

2. Once boiling, add the baking soda, stir, and then simmer for 5 to 10 minutes.

3. Using a wooden spoon, scrape the burnt-on bits from the bottom of the pot.

4. Remove from heat, rinse, and then dry with a kitchen towel.

CARPET CLEANER

While we all have household duties we find undesirable—my list is topped off with putting away the laundry and unloading the dishwasher—there's a yin for every yang. Crowning the list of housework that I *love* is vacuuming. There's something about maneuvering a big, noisy machine to suck up microscopic dust, Cheerios, and everything in between that makes me feel powerful, like a housework superhero. Plus, I find the marks that remain on the carpet once I've finished vacuuming to be endlessly satisfying. Proof that I've cleaned something! Which is why I don't really mind it when I encounter a smell, spill, dirt, or stain on my carpet, because after I give it the right baking soda treatment, I get to tie on my superhero cape and annihilate the mess!

For Odor Control

For 1 use

1–2 cups baking soda, depending on size of area to be cleaned

1. Vacuum the carpet to remove dust, debris, and pet hair.

2. Sprinkle an even layer of baking soda over the carpet.

3. Allow the baking soda to absorb odors for several hours, ideally overnight.

4. In the morning, vacuum up the powder and enjoy a fresher-smelling carpet!

Continued

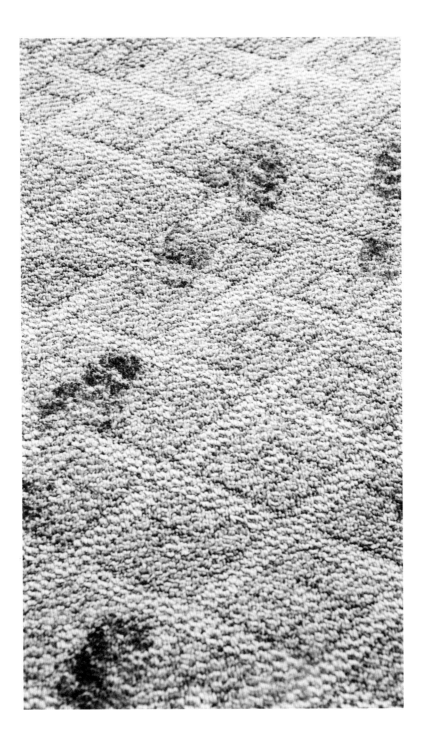

For Red Wine Stains

For 1 use

2 tablespoons baking soda

⅓ cup water

1. As soon as a spill occurs, use paper towels to blot—don't rub—as much wine as possible.

2. Pour cold water over the spill to dilute the stain; blot again with paper towels.

3. Combine baking soda and water to make a paste, then apply it to the soiled carpet, very gently massaging it into the carpet fibers.

4. Allow the paste to dry completely, then vacuum the residue.

For Urine "Accidents" (Pets or Small Humans)

For 1 use

⅛ to ¼ cup distilled white vinegar

⅛ to ¼ cup baking soda

1. Pour enough vinegar over the affected area to completely saturate the stain, being careful not to create a puddle.

2. Sprinkle baking soda over the wet vinegar; allow it to dry for several hours, ideally overnight.

3. Once dry, vacuum up the baking soda.

For General Spot Cleaning

For 1 use

1 teaspoon liquid dish soap

1 tablespoon distilled white vinegar

1 cup warm water

1 teaspoon baking soda

1. Working over a sink, combine dish soap, vinegar, and warm water in a spray bottle. With the top of the spray bottle close by, add the baking soda, and then quickly screw on the top to trap in the foam.

2. Spray the soiled area liberally with the carpet-cleaning solution, then gently rub with a cloth or paper towel.

3. Continue gently rubbing and blotting with the towel to completely remove the stain.

4. Allow carpet to dry. (You don't technically need to vacuum the carpet once dry, but who's stopping you?!)

LAUNDRY

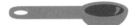

LAUNDRY AND FABRIC CARE WITH BAKING SODA

DEODORIZING "SNEAKER CREATURES"

We are an active family—that's the good news. My husband and I exercise at home and at the gym. The kids are in constant motion, running around indoors and outside, at home, at school, and on the playground. The only downside is a shoe rack full of pungent footwear! Rather than resort to storing four pairs of sneakers in hermetically sealed containers, I freshen them regularly with baking soda. This craft/deodorizer does a great job of keeping the family's athletic shoes smelling fresh—and if you have kids, they'll love helping you make them. Hats off to those dealing with teenage boy shoes. I think you, especially, will find this odor control trick to be a game-changer!

Makes 2 creatures

2 socks (new, old—doesn't matter)

2 cups baking soda

2 rubber bands

2 (6-inch) ribbons or string

Markers, buttons, felt, sequins, etc., and glue for decorating (optional)

1. Fill each sock with 1 cup baking soda.

2. Secure with a rubber band.

3. Tie ribbon around rubber band, then cut off any extra material at the cuff area.

4. Use felt, markers, buttons, googly eyes, sequins, etc. to decorate your creature.

5. Place sneaker creatures in shoes and leave overnight for fresh-smelling kicks.

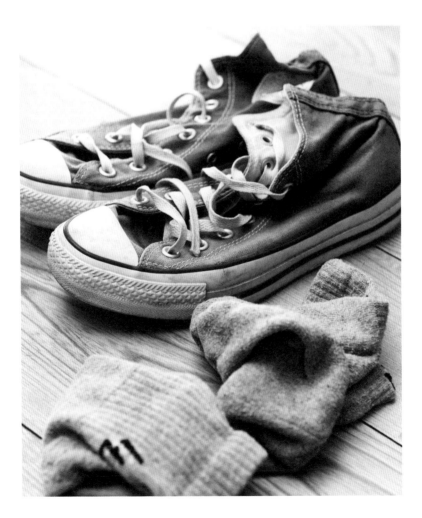

CLOTHING DE-STINKER

While gym sweat and general B.O. may first come to mind when you consider the dilemma of smelly clothes, there are a plethora of other stubborn odors that can seep into fabric and attempt to hang on for dear life, even after laundering. Fortunately, baking soda can bust through any stench from smoke to mildew to must and whatever else you've got stinking up your wardrobe (spit up, gasoline, fish . . .). Use this easy method to get the stink out for good.

For 1 use

½ cup baking soda
½ cup distilled white vinegar

1. Add laundry to the washing machine, being careful not to overfill.

2. Add baking soda directly into the machine with the clothing.

3. Fill the fabric softener tray with vinegar.

4. Wash as you normally would—no detergent.

5. Dry as usual. Sniff profusely. Unabashed.

FABRIC SOFTENER

If, like me, you have hard water where you live, you have probably found that it leaves your linens and clothes feeling a little rough. Or, perhaps, like me, you have sensitive skin and can't use fabric softener, because of the itchiness. Or maybe you just prefer to go au natural in the laundry zone, using only products with ingredients you can identify and pronounce. Well, I've got good news for you and you and all the rest of you, too! Making all-natural, non-irritating fabric softener crystals is incredibly easy to do—and the stuff really works! Double or triple the recipe and, depending on how much laundry your household produces, you should be set for a good long time. Plus, you'll be able to walk around town bragging about how you made *crystals*. How many people are gonna be able to say that at the next dinner party you go to? Not many, my friend. That's all you.

For 5 to 10 uses

2 cups coarse sea salt or kosher salt
20 to 30 drops essential oil(s) of your choice
½ cup baking soda

1. In a large bowl or storage container, combine salt and essential oil. Stir thoroughly.

2. Add baking soda and mix well.

3. Store in a container with a tight-fitting lid.

4. To use: Add ¼ to ½ cup to the wash at the same time as the laundry detergent.

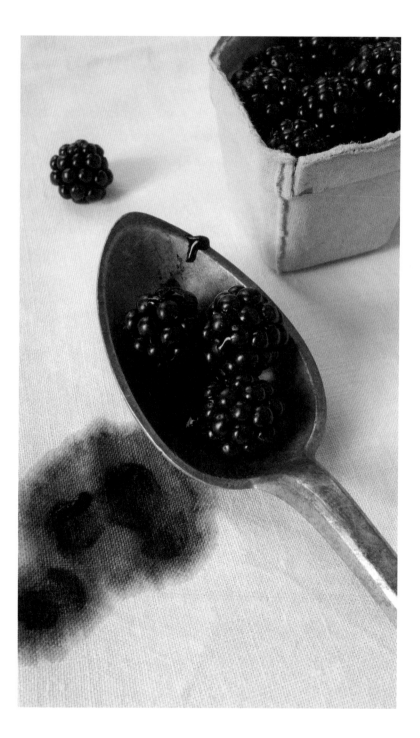

VINTAGE LINEN CLEANER

Giggle if you want, but The Royal Laundry of England is a real thing and it's where they wash the clothes and linens of all the princes, princesses, and, of course, The Queen. I imagine it to be a place where warm water and hard work are preferred over Wisk or Spray 'n Wash. I heard once about an interview that took place with the person in charge there (The Royal Launderer?) who explained that the Queen's tablecloths were never *washed*, but rather spot cleaned for stains. He purportedly said, with a totally straight face, that they used . . . wait for it . . . SPIT! I can't say one way or another what gets spilled at Buckingham Palace, but I'm confident that the spittle technique for cleaning linens would probably not work in my house, although I'm certain my kids would be happy to give it a try. Meanwhile, I *can* say that if you have fine, vintage, or antique linens that have become, dirty, dulled, and even yellowed, there is a way to restore them—no Royal Spitter required. Try this antique dealers' trick to make old bed and table linens look almost as good as new.

For 1 use

¼ cup Epsom salt
½ cup baking soda

1. Place stained or yellowed linens in a very large pot of water.

2. Add Epsom salt and baking soda.

Continued

3. Bring the pot to a boil on the stove. Remove from heat and stir.

4. Allow the linens to soak for several hours, stirring occasionally.

5. For severely soiled or yellowed linens, repeat process one or more times.

6. Discard baking soda solution and rinse fabric thoroughly in cool water.

7. To dry, hang the pieces on a clothesline outdoors or lay flat on the grass. Sunlight acts as a natural brightener. Do not put in a clothes dryer.

Tip: For very stubborn stains, try this: Dampen the spot to be cleaned. Pour lemon juice through the stain and sprinkle generously with salt, then place in the sun for several hours. When dry, rinse thoroughly to remove all traces of the lemon and salt. Hang or lie flat to air dry, ideally in the sun.

WHITENING AND BRIGHTENING LAUNDRY BOOSTER

Lest you think that the only way to get "whiter whites and brighter brights" is to enhance your laundry detergent with something that comes out of a plastic tub emblazoned with sparkling rainbows and a name like *Kapow!*, think again. Adding just a little bit of baking soda to your regular laundry detergent

Continued

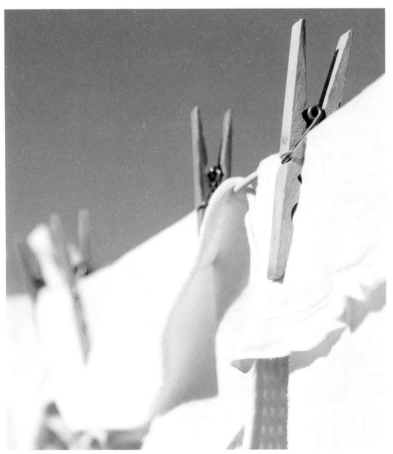

will give you bright, white, fresh, and clean laundry without any weird or harsh chemicals. In addition to balancing the pH in the wash, which results in clean and dazzling clothes, baking soda softens the water, allowing you to use less detergent—a bonus for the Earth and your wallet! Plus, it increases the potency of bleach, so you can cut down there, too. In summary, to get the best-looking laundry on the block, skip the "color-safe bleach" and commercially produced "laundry booster" and, instead, pump it up yourself!

For 1 use

¼ to ½ cup baking soda (½ cup baking soda for top-loading machines; ¼ cup for front-loaders)

1. Add baking soda along with your regular liquid laundry detergent at the start of the wash cycle. Use less baking soda for smaller loads. Wash as usual.

2. If you are using a powder detergent, add the baking soda to the washing machine during the rinse cycle.

STAIN REMOVER

Baking soda is great and all, but sometimes it can be such a showoff. Take stain removal, for example. Sure, baking soda can handle most stains with one hand tied behind its back, but . . . I mean, seriously, the ego! You've got a red wine stain? Baking soda thinks that's an easy one. Blood? Baking soda's all, "yeah, whatever . . . " Grass? Baking soda rolls its eyes. We get it, OK? You're good at removing stains. Sheesh!

Here are some common and (I hope) not-so-common stains that can be tackled, treated, and kicked to the curb with baking soda.

Lipstick

For 1 use

3 teaspoons baking soda
¼ teaspoon distilled white vinegar

1. Gently blot the lipstick stain with a soft cloth or tissue.

2. Apply 2 teaspoons baking soda directly to the stain and, using a toothbrush, gently scrub the affected area until it has absorbed much of the oil and pigment. The baking soda will become tinted. Rinse the toothbrush thoroughly to remove all traces of lipstick.

Continued

3. Brush away the tinted baking soda and discard. Add remaining teaspoon of baking soda to the stain. Sprinkle the white vinegar over the baking soda and allow the mixture to foam.

4. With the clean toothbrush, gently scrub the affected area again until the stain is gone, and then launder as usual.

Red Wine

For 1 use

1 to 2 tablespoons baking soda
¼ cup distilled white vinegar
Club soda

1. Dab the stain with cloth or paper towels to absorb as much wine as possible. Do not rub!

2. Sprinkle baking soda over the stain and allow it to sit for several minutes—it will change from red to pale grey.

3. Pour vinegar over the stain and rinse with club soda.

4. Once the stain is removed, launder as usual.

Vomit

For 1 use

¼ to ⅓ cup baking soda
1 tablespoon distilled white vinegar or lemon juice

1. Scrape any solids off the fabric.

2. Spread the fabric on a flat surface and dampen the stain with warm water. Apply enough baking soda to cover the stain by about ¼ inch.

3. Pour vinegar or lemon juice over the stain. Allow the mixture to foam.

4. Using a toothbrush, gently scrub the affected area until the stain appears to be gone.

5. Rinse clothing with warm water, and then machine wash as usual.

Blood

For 1 use

1 tablespoon shampoo or liquid dish soap
Cold water
2 tablespoons baking soda

Continued

1. Pre-treat old or set-in blood stains with shampoo or liquid dish soap.

2. Soak the stained garment in cold water for 10 to 30 minutes.

3. After soaking, pour baking soda onto the stain and scrub with a toothbrush.

4. Wash the garment as you normally would in the washing machine.

Sweat

For 1 use

4 tablespoons baking soda
¼ cup warm water

1. Run the stained area under water.

2. Combine baking soda and warm water to make a paste.

3. Spread paste on the stained garment, then gently rub the cloth together.

4. Allow the paste to sit for 30 to 60 minutes.

5. Rinse and machine-wash as usual.

Grass

For 1 use

1 tablespoon baking soda

1 tablespoon hydrogen peroxide

1. Combine baking soda and hydrogen peroxide to create a paste.

2. Spread the paste over the stain.

3. Soak for 10 minutes, then launder as usual.

Note: While very effective, this combo can discolor fabric, so don't leave it on for too long.

WASHING MACHINE CLEANER

I lived in New York City for many years, where, like most apartment dwellers, I didn't have my own laundry machines. The trick to surviving this particular way of life is to NEVER let yourself think about when (or worse—whether) the machine you've just used was last cleaned. If you've never used a communal laundry room or washed your clothes at a laundromat, you might not have given much thought to the process of cleaning a washing machine. I mean, soap goes in there regularly, so it's probably clean enough, right? Not so much. Consider what goes into a washing machine: bits of food, dead skin cells, sweat, dirt (and if you have a baby, there is *other* organic matter, if you know what I mean . . .). All of that can get caught in the crevices and hard-to-reach places of a washer. And want to know what grows in perpetually dark, damp, and warm environments? Mildew and mold, that's what! Plus, laundry detergents and water deposits can build up, which are good for neither your machine nor your laundry. In short, washing machines need to be cleaned on the reg. And here's how:

For 1 use

¼ cup baking soda
¼ cup water
2 cups distilled white vinegar

1. Combine baking soda and water in a small bowl.

2. For front-loading machines, add the baking soda mixture to the detergent container of your machine and pour the

vinegar into the tub. For top-loading machines, add it all to the tub.

3. Turn your washer to the hottest temperature setting. Close the door and set the machine to run a regular load.

4. Use a damp sponge or rag to rub around the opening of the machine, removing any mold or remaining residue. Rinse clean with plain water.

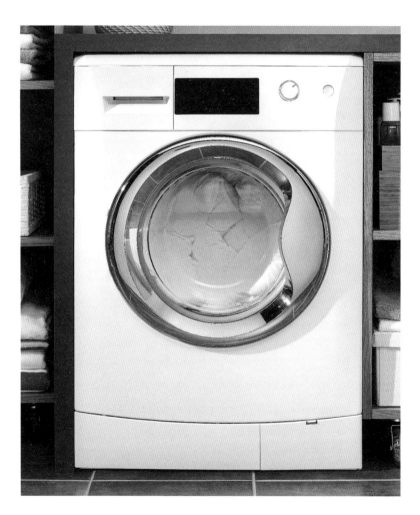

SUEDE CLEANER

Anyone who has ever owned anything suede knows what a production it can be to keep clean. Elvis Presley sang about it: "You can do anything / but stay off of my blue suede shoes." Yeah, because he *knew*. I bet he loved those shoes because they were 1) incredibly durable and 2) always fashionable. If you're in the same boat as Elvis and his blue suede shoes (or me and my pink suede hobo bag), rest assured that there's a shortcut to keeping your suede goods soft, chic, and tip-top. Baking soda rids suede of stains, scuffs, and other unsightly blemishes so you can get on with your fabulous life. Give it a try.

For 1 use

Distilled white vinegar
Baking soda

1. Wipe away surface dirt and dust with a clean, soft cloth.

2. To clean liquid stains: Soak up the spill with a paper towel as quickly as possible, applying firm pressure. Using a clean towel, dampened slightly with white vinegar, dab at the stain to remove. Allow it to dry.

3. To clean grease or oil stains: Blot the area with a cloth or paper towel to remove as much of the stain as possible, then cover with baking soda and leave for several hours.

4. Once stains have been removed and suede is dry, sprinkle a light dusting of baking soda over the surface of the suede, then buff thoroughly with a suede brush or soft toothbrush to refresh the nap.

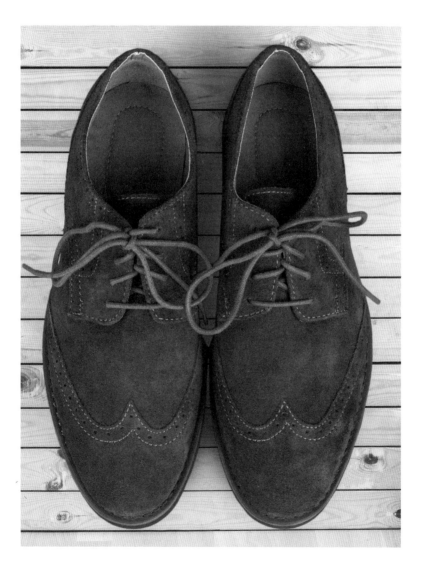

GENTLE WASHING POWDER FOR BABY CLOTHES

When I was pregnant with my first kid, I logged enough hours researching baby-related topics to earn a doctorate degree in Newborn Preparedness. I'd gone cross-eyed reading about car seats, cribs, bassinets, breastfeeding, safety gates, burp cloths, diapers, and baby food. I'd gathered safety ratings, reviews, warnings, and advice from doctors, relatives, veteran moms, police, consumer groups, NIH, and the CDC. The funny thing is, in addition to being crazy-making (thanks, hormones), all that "knowledge" didn't actually prepare me for what happens once a new baby arrives. Take laundry, for example. Sure, I knew that we needed to wash all of our daughter's clothing and linens in extremely gentle detergent to protect her delicate, new skin, but I had NO idea how freaking often we'd be doing that!! The sheer volume of laundry generated by that teeny little peeing, pooping, spitting-up bundle of joy was staggering, and nothing could have prepared us for how quickly we'd go through a box of fragrance-free, dye-free, everything-free detergent. A few weeks in, however, something I'd learned in my Internet travels *did* manage to bubble up from my sleep-deprived brain: I could quickly and easily make my own detergent with only the most basic ingredients—no questionable additives such as sodium laurel sulfate or other possible irritants. It's green, it's safe, and it's cheap. Not quite as life changing as bringing home a new baby, but it's up there . . .

Continued

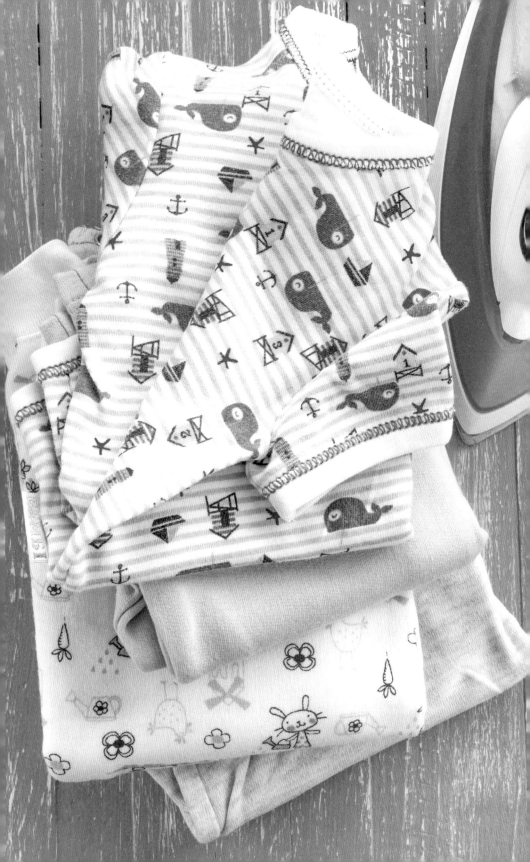

Makes about 15 cups (or 60 loads, which juuust might get you through that first month of new parenthood. Ha.)

8 cups baking soda

6 cups Super Washing Soda (all-natural product found in the laundry aisle, also known as "washing soda" or "soda ash")

2 bars castile soap, grated

1. Combine all the ingredients together and store in an airtight container.

2. Optional step: Pulse the grated soap in a blender or food processor along with some of the baking soda to achieve a finer soap powder.

3. To use, add ¼ to ⅛ cup detergent to baby's laundry, depending on load size.

TOWEL REVIVER

It's not easy being a towel. All that dirt and oil, hard water, and friction can really beat a textile down. If you've found that your towels have become rough, less absorbent, or otherwise lackluster over time, offer a little TLC in the form of baking soda to keep them looking and feeling their best. Baking soda helps loosen up fibers and remove chemical residue and grime, thus restoring your towels to their formerly soft and fluffy

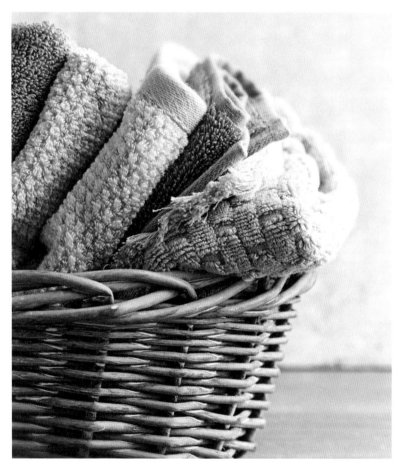

Continued

selves. Plus, baking soda naturally eliminates musty or mildewy odors that result from leaving damp towels lying around for too long. A word to the wise: Don't put too many towels in your washer at once. A too-big load = not enough room to properly rinse your towels in the washer or properly fluff them in the dryer. For most machines, two or three bath towels at a time, along with hand towels and washcloths, will probably give you the best result.

For 1 use

½ cup baking soda

1. Set washer temperature to warm setting.

2. Add baking soda directly to washer along with your regular detergent.

3. Wash and dry as usual.

CARE FOR DELICATE CLOTHING

I'm going to admit right here and now that I am a person who washes her bras in the washing machine and sometimes, when I forget to hang them up, dries them the dryer—*gasp!* I know! I'm an absolute barbarian! Now, in my defense and with apologies to my husband, I'm not exactly sporting delicate La Perla lingerie these days. If I were spending more on my bras, I'd probably wash them by hand. And if I washed my bras (and swimsuits and other delicates) by hand, I'd certainly do so using this lovely baking soda method.

For 1 use

Cold water
¼ cup baking soda
A few drops of essential oil, if desired

1. Fill a sink with cold water and add baking soda and essential oil, if using.

2. Soak your delicates in the mixture for about 15 minutes.

3. Rinse with cool water, then hang dry.

SMELLY HAMPER REMEDY

When we moved into our house a few years ago, I decided I wanted a "pretty" hamper for our bedroom. We'd always used the pop-up mesh kind, which is practical for lugging dirty clothes down to the laundry room and is breathable, an attribute whose importance I would come to appreciate later. But our old hamper (hot pink mesh, just to give you the full picture) couldn't compete on the looks scale with the stylish, ink blue, lidded hamper I'd found to perfectly conceal our dirty laundry while complementing the moody gray paint on our bedroom walls. The problem was, the not-so-cute dirty sock smell our beautiful hamper began to emit after a few months, even when it was empty. There was no way I was going back to an unsightly hamper situation. I'd committed to style over function, so my only choice was to attack the stink head on. I considered simply keeping a box of baking soda nearby and sprinkling a bit directly into the hamper and onto the dirty clothes every once in a while, but that seemed like adding more work to a chore I already found tedious. So, if you're like me and pink mesh isn't your thing, try this odor buffer to keep smells at bay until you *finally* get around to doing the laundry.

For 1 use

¼ cup baking soda
Paper coffee filter

1. Add baking soda to the coffee filter.

2. Fold it in half and staple or tape it shut.

3. Place in the bottom of the hamper, where it will absorb odors.

4. Replace with a new one as odors return, usually every month or so.

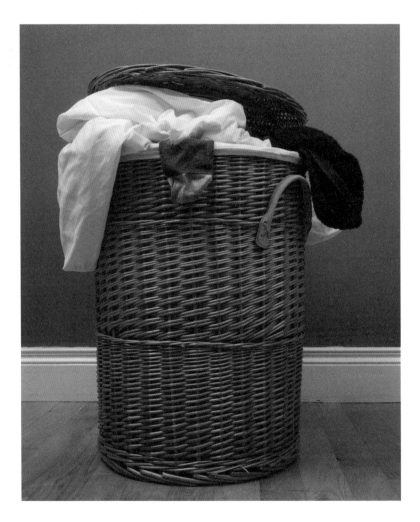

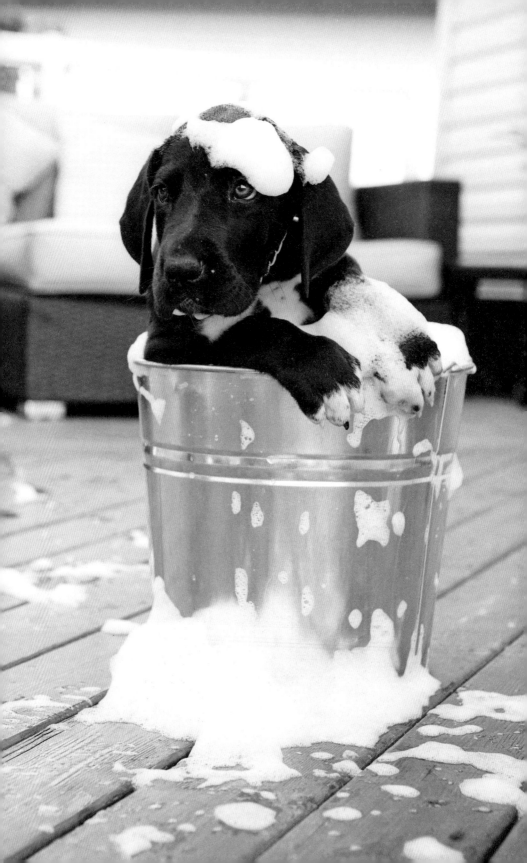

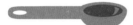

OUTDOOR USES FOR BAKING SODA

GRILL CLEANER

In the summer, when the weather is nice, outdoor grillin' and chillin' is definitely what I'm about. But there is truly nothing worse than being pumped about grilling only to open the lid of your grill and discover dirty grates. I try—really I do—to remember to clean them right after I finish cooking, but sometimes I forget. The resulting mess can be tough to tackle. Sometimes, even with heating up the grill for a good 15 minutes, and then scrubbing the hot grates with a steel brush, some residue (and neglect) remains. For reasons such as this, it's worth giving your grill a more thorough scrub a few times a year to ensure that you have a safe, top-performing, good-food-makin' grill.

For 1 use

¼ cup baking soda
¼ cup water

1. Combine baking soda and water to make a paste.

2. Apply the paste directly to the grill grate, scrub with a wire brush, and let dry for 15 minutes.

3. Wipe down the grates with a dry cloth, then place over hot coals (or over high heat on a gas grill) for at least 15 minutes to burn off any residue before placing food on top.

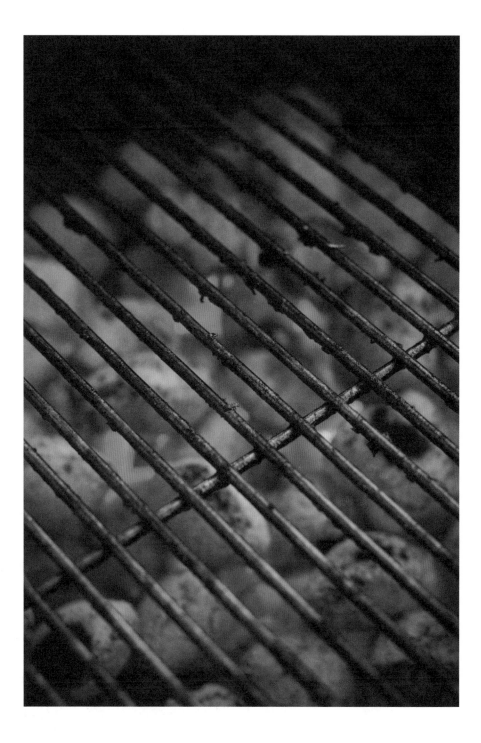

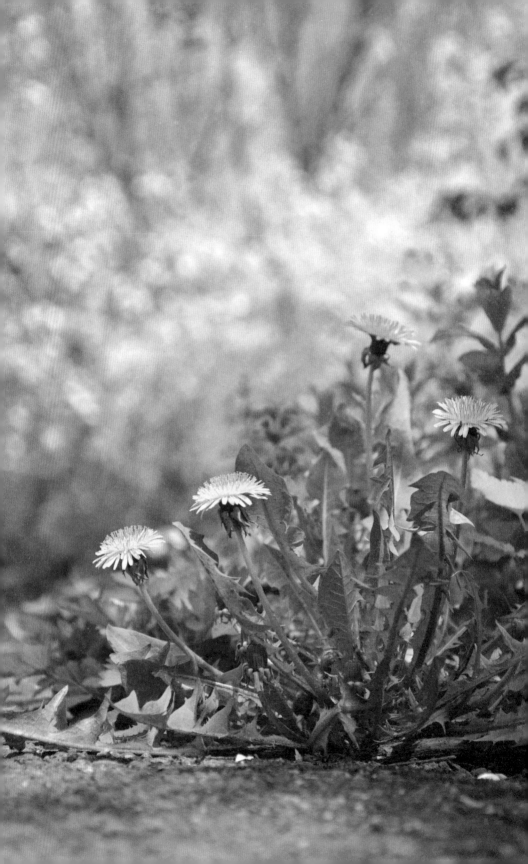

WEED KILLER

Here's something I've learned in my attempts to conquer suburbia: Gardening is a boatload of work. It is not the easy and relaxing past-time I expected it to be. Gratifying? Yes. But, effortless? Nuh-uh! Keeping a landscaped yard looking attractive and non-junglelike involves making sure the grass is mowed, the edges are trimmed, the plants are watered, the shrubs are pruned, and the beds are weeded—*record scratch*. Weeding. That's the part where I start to shut down. I can convince myself to a certain degree that letting weeds grow in the backyard somehow contributes to a dynamic "native plant landscape," but when it comes to the brick walkway leading to our front door, there's no escaping it. The pervasive and persistent weeds that show up between the cracks are unsightly and (I'm guessing) damaging to the bricks. And you can't pull those buggers out. I've tried. You have to kill them. But how do you do that without using dangerous pesticides? The answer is so simple, it's almost silly—boiling water and baking soda. The combination zaps pesky weeds that lurk in the cracks of walkways, driveways, sidewalks, and patios completely and quickly, leaving you with one less outdoor chore to avoid.

For 1 use

Continued

Baking soda

Boiling water

1. Put a pot or kettle of tap water on the stove and bring to a boil.

2. Pour the hot water over the weeds you wish to kill.

3. Sprinkle handfuls of baking soda directly onto the areas where weeds have been treated with boiling water, sweeping excess baking soda into the cracks and crevices.

4. Wait a day or two for results, then reapply treatment on areas where live weeds remain.

Note: This treatment should only be used in places where you want no plant growth (such as driveways, sidewalk cracks, underneath decks and patio blocks, around the foundation of the house, etc.), because it kills everything. *Everything.*

WINDOW CLEANER

Dirty windows are one of those houseworky things that I tend to ignore as long as I possibly can—usually until something like the following conversation takes place:

Me: Babe, where'd you put the *really good* umbrella? I need to take it today.

Husband: Really? An umbrella?

Me: Yeah, it's about to rain. Look at the clouds!

Husband: [opens front door] Uh, looks pretty sunny out there. No clouds.

Me: Then why do I keep expecting to see John Cusack holding a boom box over his head in the pouring rain every time I look out the window?

Husband: Mostly because you love '80s romantic comedies, but also because we need to wash the windows. By the way, I don't think it's raining during that scene in *Say Anything*.

Me: Yeah, but you knew what I was talking about.

Husband: [hands me the baking soda, humming Peter Gabriel's "In Your Eyes"]

For 1 use

½ to 1 cup baking soda, or more depending on number of windows

1 to 2 cups water, plus more for rinsing

1 to 2 cups distilled white vinegar

Continued

1. Dampen a cloth or paper towel with plain water, then sprinkle with baking soda. Gently scrub the window to completely remove any visible dirt.

2. Dip a clean cloth or paper towel in plain warm water and wipe the window to remove any residual baking soda.

3. Combine equal parts water and vinegar in a spray bottle. Spray the window with the mixture and quickly wipe dry with clean cloth or paper towels.

4. Once dry, buff the window with a soft chamois cloth, crumpled newspaper, or a clean chalkboard eraser to enhance shine and to remove streaks.

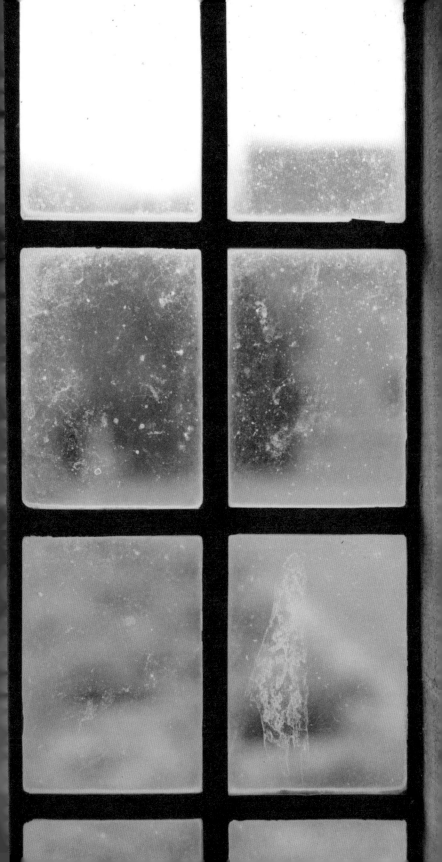

ALUMINUM AND VINYL SIDING CLEANER

Many homeowners live under the (mistaken) impression that the only way to effectively clean the exterior of their home is with a pressure washer. While I confess to having daydreamed about using a power washer to clean all kinds of stuff around my house and yard (doesn't that sound simultaneously fun and satisfying??), it's not actually necessary when it comes to cleaning the outside of your house. When your vinyl or aluminum siding starts to go mucky, whip up this no-pressure homemade baking soda solution to keep up your curb appeal. You *can* use this cleaner with a power washer or by simply following the hand-washing directions below.

For 1 use

4 tablespoons liquid dish soap

¼ cup baking soda

2 cups warm water

4 tablespoons distilled white vinegar

1. In a bucket, combine liquid dish soap and baking soda. Stir until the baking soda is dissolved.

2. Add the warm water to the dish soap and baking soda mixture. Stir gently to avoid forming bubbles.

3. Add the vinegar. Mix thoroughly.

4. To use: Using a soft, damp towel wipe the solution onto the siding. Rinse with warm water to remove any residue.

Note: If you're cleaning your siding by hand, avoid using a scrub brush, steel wool pad, or any stiff-bristled brush that could scratch or tear the vinyl.

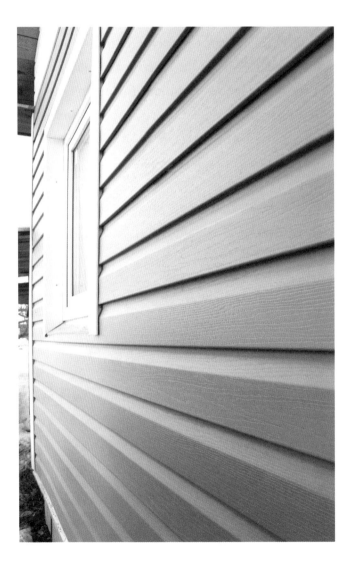

LAWN FURNITURE CLEANER

Who doesn't love relaxing in the backyard on a perfect day? Sunny, but not blazing, a gentle breeze blowing, perhaps a glass of iced tea in hand. . . . Sounds lovely to me. But getting ready to sink into a chaise that's caked with dirt, dust, and some kind of greenish film that can only be classified as "outdoor gunk" kills the relaxation before it starts. Routine cleaning is the key to keeping outdoor furniture in tip-top (non-gross) shape. For best results, clean your outdoor furniture with this solution two to four times a year: once at the beginning of summer, once at the end of summer, and—if you're really on top of things—a couple of times in between.

For 1 use

1 cup baking soda
3 gallons warm water

1. Mix baking soda with water in a 3-gallon bucket.

2. Using a cloth or sponge, wipe down furniture with baking soda solution.

3. Rinse furniture with a garden hose and either towel dry your furniture or allow it to air dry in the sunshine.

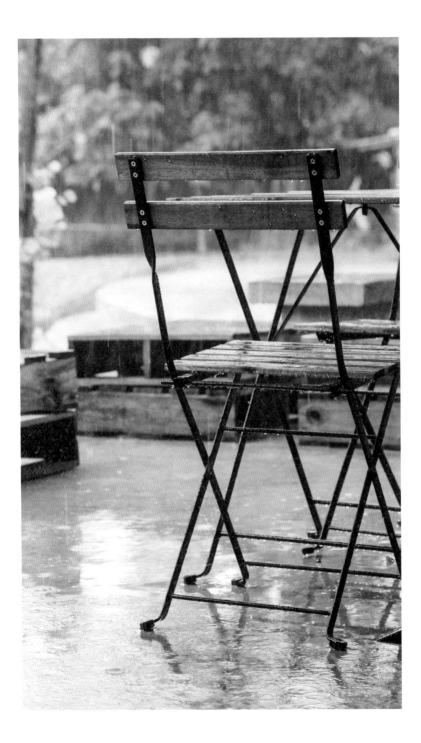

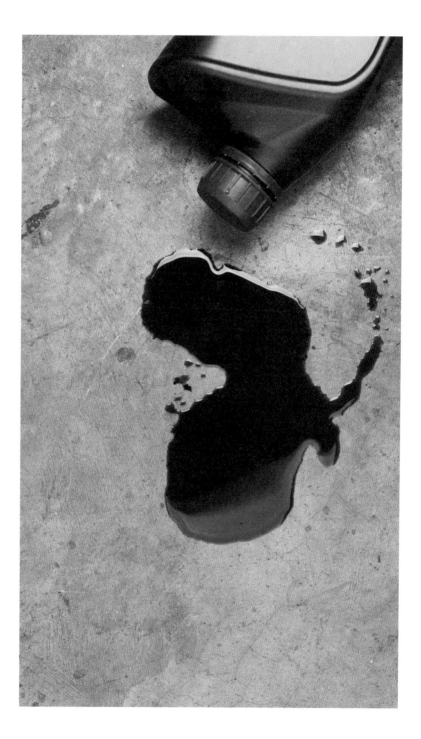

The Baking Soda Companion

CLEANUP FOR GARAGE OIL SPILLS

My garage floor had seen better days. Every time I pulled my car in, I looked at my poor stained floor and sighed a helpless little sigh. I mean, I know it's where the car goes and all, but did it really have to look like the floor of the parking structure at the mall? Yet, for the longest time, I didn't actually do anything about it (other than the sigh), because I was convinced that my only options were to paint it (which seemed kind of ridiculous) or replace it entirely (which seemed even more ridiculous), and I wasn't even sure those were viable options. Then, finally, I started to wonder if I could clean it. *Duh*. I knew the stains were old and I wasn't 100 percent sure what they were, but I assumed I was looking at grease, maybe paint... probably nothing a little baking soda couldn't take care of. So I decided I would give it a shot, and HOLY MOLY was I surprised at how well it turned out! My garage floor looks like a million bucks, and not only did it take me about 30 minutes to complete, but the whole thing cost me about $2 in supplies.

For 1 use

1 to 2 cups baking soda
1 cup distilled white vinegar
½ cup laundry detergent
2 gallons hot water

Continued

1. Apply baking soda directly to grease stains and allow it to sit for several minutes to absorb the grease.

2. Meanwhile, in a large bucket, combine vinegar, laundry detergent, and hot water.

3. Pour the cleaning solution onto the floor and, using a scrub brush or a stiff shop broom, scrub mixture to get it deep down into the texture of the concrete.

4. Rinse your floor with a hose on full blast to remove dirt and detergent.

5. Allow the floor to air dry. If necessary, repeat the process several times to remove all stains.

PH BALANCER FOR POOLS AND SPAS

I do not now nor have I ever owned or maintained a pool or spa. However, I am forever amazed by the endless uses for baking soda, so I have to include this gem for those of you who do. As I've learned, keeping a balanced pH is a critical part of swimming pool maintenance. Not only does the right pH protect the metal fittings and the walls of the pool, the right pH range is what makes swimming in the water enjoyable instead of an itchy, prickly experience. The correct range for a swimming pool is a pH of 7.2 to 7.8. Baking soda can be used in pool and hot tub water to adjust pH upward if it dips low. It also helps prevent the pH from moving out of the desirable range. (P.S. If you happen to live near me, an invitation to swim is all the thanks I need for dropping this bit of knowledge!)

For 1 to 2 uses

9 to 15 pounds baking soda

1. Check the pH of your pool water. If it has dropped below 7.2, add 9 pounds of baking soda per 10,000 gallons of water to raise the pH.

2. Check the pH again in a day. If it has not stabilized and/ or drops below 7.2 again, add another 6 pounds of baking soda per 10,000 gallons of water.

3. Your pH should remain between 7.2 and 7.8 for several weeks.

CAR WASH SOLUTION

Shortly after we moved to the suburbs, I realized my daughter had never been to a car wash. So as not to deprive her of the sudsy, sloshing fun of driving through, I decided to take her one morning. Just as I'd hoped, she loved the experience and I wanted to capture her squeals of delight on camera. But it was dark in the car under all those brushes and foam, so I reached up to turn on the interior light in order to shoot a better video, but instead of hitting *that* button, I hit the one that opens the sun roof. The resulting video captures my squeals, rather than hers, and then our collective maniacal laughter as I scrambled to quickly close the roof while a pile of soapsuds collected on my drenched head. As much as I like to entertain my kids, I don't plan to repeat that performance. Thankfully, pulling on their bathing suits and washing the car in our driveway entertains them equally. Here's the solution we use to get the Family Truckster sparkling.

For 1 use

¼ cup baking soda
¼ cup liquid dish soap
Water

1. Pour baking soda into a gallon-size jug, then add dish soap and enough water to fill the jug almost to the top.

2. Screw on the cap, shake well, and store the concentrate for later use.

3. When it comes time to wash the car, shake the jug vigorously, then pour 1 cup of cleaner base into a 2-gallon water pail.

4. Fill the pail with warm water, stir to mix, and your homemade cleaning solution is ready to use. Spraying each other with the hose is optional, but encouraged.

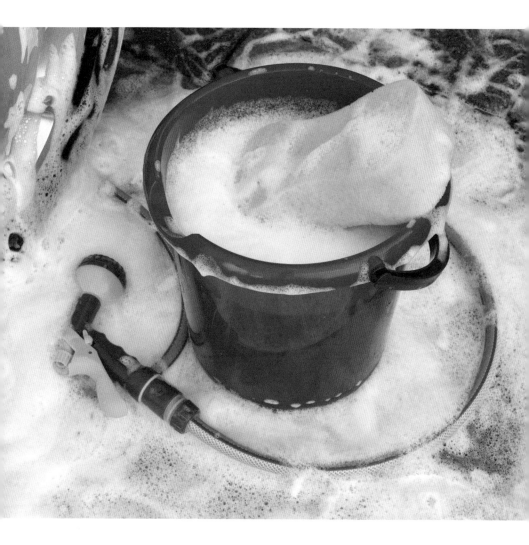

COMPOST BIN ODOR REDUCER

When I finally decided to start composting, I'd already spent a lot of time thinking about it. After we'd left the city, I had fewer and fewer excuses for not doing it. We had the space, we would be sending less waste to landfills, our struggling-but-brimming-with-potential garden would surely become amazing, and we'd likely learn something from the process. The concept, while somewhat intimidating, seemed like it would be satisfying and felt like the right thing to do. I worried about the smell, though. Would my house stink? My yard? As it turns out, composting isn't a big deal at all, and if you're doing it right, odor isn't usually an issue. We keep a small bin in our kitchen that we dump into a larger heap in our backyard when it gets full. Most of the time there's no smell, although we do occasionally find that the indoor bin can develop somewhat of a funk, something that I've learned is easily overcome with the help of baking soda, which reduces the acidity of compost. To keep your compost smells at bay, try this technique:

Makes 1 packet

1 old sock
¼ to 1 cup baking soda, depending on the size of your bin

1. Fill the sock with baking soda, then close securely with twine, a rubber band, or a twist tie.

2. Place in the bottom of the compost bin.

3. Replace every 1 to 3 months.

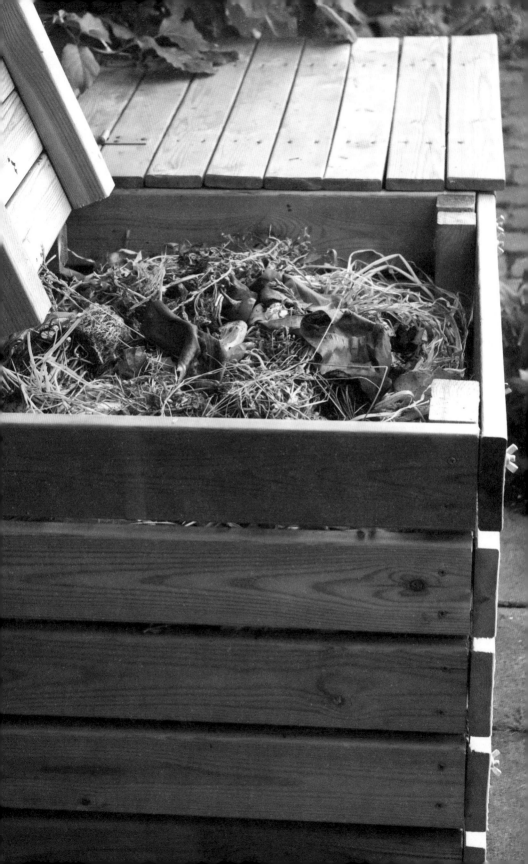

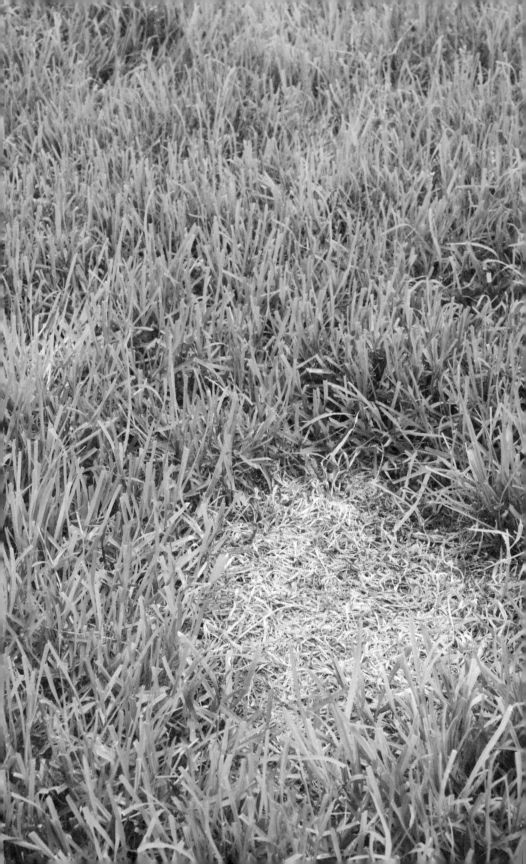

RX FOR GRASS THAT PETS LOVE

Growing up, our family's dog, Senorita Bandita (Bandi, for short), loved to frolic in our backyard. She was a sweet dog, but she'd flunked out of obedience school, partly for her lack of social skills, so she spent a lot of time on her own behind our house. Frolicking. Alas, with happy dog frolicking comes happy dog peeing. And with happy dog peeing comes not-so-happy brown spots on a lawn. Dog pee, which is heavy in acid and nitrogen, actually burns the grass, which is unsightly, to say the least. There are several chemical solutions to this very common problem but I recommend a natural approach. Pouring a baking soda mixture directly on burn spots neutralizes the intensity of the ammonia and nitrogen that are in the urine and restores the scorched grass to green beauty. It's effective for the lawn and healthy for frolicking dogs, who might otherwise ingest toxic lawn chemicals when they lick their paws.

For 1 use

2 tablespoons baking soda
1 gallon water

1. Dissolve baking soda in a gallon of water.

2. Pour the baking soda mixture over the spot where the pet has urinated. The baking soda will neutralize the ammonia and nitrogen present in the urine, preventing the grass from turning brown.

TOMATO PLANT SWEETENER

Maybe it's that they come in a rainbow of colors or that every variety is distinctive, but there's something about homegrown tomatoes that makes me swoon. When they're in season, I can't get enough of their sweet deliciousness. But, contrary to popular belief, not all tomato plants give off sweet tomatoes—even homegrown ones. The actual flavor of a tomato comes from a combination of the plant chemistry and variables that are present in their growing location such as air temperature, soil type, and the amount of sun and rain in a growing season. Of course, some of those factors are within your control and some are not. You may not have power over the weather, but you *can* treat your garden soil to encourage ideal tomato-ness! When setting the scene for your next bumper crop of sweet and juicy tomatoes, try adding a bit of baking soda to the soil. It lowers the acidity level, giving you crops that are more sweet than tart. Here's how:

Treats 1 plant

¼ cup baking soda per tomato plant

1. When tomatoes begin to appear and are about 1 inch in diameter, lightly sprinkle baking soda on the soil around each plant, being careful not to get the baking soda on the plant itself.

2. Repeat when the tomatoes are about halfway grown.

Continued

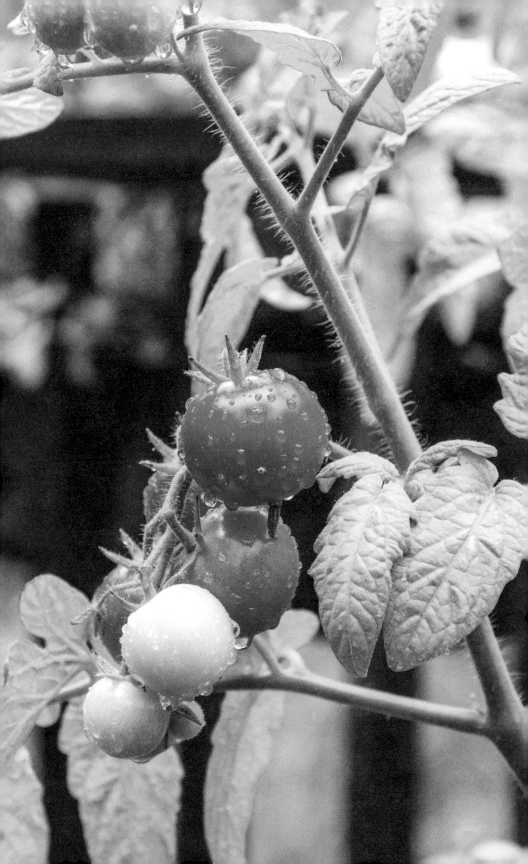

5 MORE USES FOR BAKING SODA IN THE GARDEN:

1. Eliminate powdery mildew: Mix 1 tablespoon baking soda, 1 gallon water, 1 tablespoon vegetable oil, and 1 tablespoon dish soap. Spray weekly on affected plants.

2. Refresh rose bushes: Water roses with 1 teaspoon baking soda, ½ teaspoon clear ammonia, and 1 teaspoon Epsom salt in a gallon of water.

3. Make a fungicide: Combine a gallon of water with 1 tablespoon baking soda, 2½ tablespoons vegetable oil, and ½ teaspoon of castile soap. Spray on the foliage of diseased plants.

4. Test your soil pH: Wet the soil and sprinkle a small amount of baking soda onto it. If the baking soda bubbles, your soil is acidic with a pH level under 5.

5. Repel garden pests: Rabbits, ants, silver fish, and roaches don't like baking soda. Sprinkle it on the perimeter of your garden to keep them away.

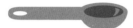

10 FUN THINGS TO DO WITH BAKING SODA

Useful as baking soda is for cooking, cleaning, and health and beauty, there's a fun side to the domestic workhorse, too! Delight and amaze your loved ones with these super cool science and craft projects that go far beyond run-of-the-mill erupting volcanoes.

Invisible Ink

Combine equal parts baking soda and water to make a paste. Dip a cotton swab, toothpick, or thin paintbrush into the mixture, then write a message on a piece of paper and let it dry completely. To decode the message, paint the paper with purple grape juice concentrate. The acid in the juice will react with the alkaline baking soda and turn the message a different color.

Ooey Gooey Slime

In a small bowl, combine ½ cup white school glue and enough liquid laundry detergent to achieve a slimy and sticky consistency, about 1 to 2 teaspoons. In another bowl, combine 1 tablespoon baking soda and 1 tablespoon water (plus a few drops of food color, if you like). Add 1 teaspoon of the baking soda/water mixture to the glue/detergent slime. Use your hands to incorporate all ingredients evenly. You'll be left with a smooth, stretchy, perfectly gross slime.

Fizzy Bath Bombs

In a large bowl, combine 1 cup baking soda, ½ cup salt, ½ cup powdered citric acid, and ¾ cup cornstarch. Set aside. In a small bowl, mix 2 tablespoons olive oil, 2 teaspoons witch hazel, 1 teaspoon vanilla extract, and 20 to 30 drops essential oil. Using your hands to mix, slowly add the wet ingredients to the dry ingredients. Working quickly, firmly pack the resulting mixture into bath bomb molds or greased muffin tins. Press in firmly and allow to dry for 24 hours or until hardened.

Air-Dry Crafting Clay

Heat 1¼ cups water, 2 cups baking soda, and 1 cup cornstarch in a pot set over medium heat. Stir the mixture constantly until it thickens and becomes the consistency of mashed potatoes. Allow it to cool, then knead until smooth and no longer sticky. Now play! Clay can be stored in an airtight container in the fridge for up to one week, or you can air-dry the finished product overnight. Once dry, creations can be painted with tempera or acrylic craft paints.

Microwave Puffy Paint

In a bowl, mix 1 cup flour, 3 teaspoons baking soda, and 1 teaspoon salt. Gradually add 1 to 1¼ cups water until you have a mixture the consistency of pancake batter. Mix in food coloring of your choice. (To make multiple colors, divide un-dyed paint into separate containers before adding food coloring.) Pour the puffy paint into squeeze bottles or re-sealable plastic baggies with one corner snipped off. Squeeze paint onto paper to create a masterpiece, then microwave on high for 30 seconds to dry and puff!

Balloon Experiment

Use a funnel to fill a plastic bottle about ¼ of the way with distilled white vinegar—empty 2-liter soda bottles work well. Place the opening of a balloon around the funnel and fill it with 2 to 3 teaspoons baking soda. Stretch the opening of the balloon to fit over the opening of the bottle, then lift the balloon up so that the baking soda drops down into the vinegar. Watch as the balloon fills with air!

Dancing Raisins

Fill a glass halfway with warm water. Add 3 heaping teaspoons baking soda. Stir to dissolve. Drop 4 to 6 raisins into the glass. Put the glass on a tray or in the sink (to catch the overflow), then top with ¼ to ½ cup distilled white vinegar. Wait for the foam to subside, then watch as the raisins eventually begin to rise and fall.

Fizzy Egg Dye

Mix 2 parts baking soda and 1 part water that has been tinted with food coloring to make a thick, colorful paste. Using a brush or cotton swabs, decorate the eggs as desired. Once eggs are completely covered in paint, drop them into a glass of distilled white vinegar. The vinegar will fizz and overflow. Remove your egg with a spoon to find it beautifully colored. Note: This experiment can get messy. To mitigate the chaos, do it over a sink or outside.

Lava Lamp

Add 3 to 4 tablespoons baking soda to the bottom of a clean, dry bottle. Shake gently to help the baking soda settle into a flat layer. Using a funnel, fill the bottle ¾ full with vegetable or baby oil, then add enough water to nearly fill the bottle. In a small bowl, combine ½ cup distilled white vinegar and 5 to 6 drops of food coloring. Using a pipette, eyedropper, or turkey baster, add 5 to 6 drops colored vinegar into the bottle. Watch what happens. Continue to add more drops of vinegar into the bottle until the bubbles stop floating to the surface. For an authentic lava lamp experience, do this experiment in a dark room and put a bright flashlight behind the bottle. And maybe put on some Pink Floyd.

Watercolor Paint

Combine 1 tablespoon distilled white vinegar and 1 tablespoon baking soda in a bowl. When the mixture stops foaming, add 1 tablespoon cornstarch and ½ teaspoon corn syrup. Stir well. Divide the mixture between containers (empty egg cartons and lids from old spice jars work well). Add a few drops of food coloring to each container and blend with a toothpick or paintbrush. Watercolors can be used immediately or left to dry into cakes.

ACKNOWLEDGMENTS

I am indebted to everyone who helped me along the long and powdery road to this book. Thank you to Sharon Bowers for your endless well of support, enthusiasm, and guidance. To Ann Treistman for saying "yes" to a book entirely about baking soda, of all things, and for the ensuing enthusiastic supervision. To Aurora Bell and the rest of the team at The Countryman Press for bringing this project to life.

To my amazing family and friends: Many of you willingly and generously became the subjects of science experiments, testing various salves, scrubs, tonics, and potions. Some of you watched my kids, others of you cheered me on, and some of you poured me wine. Thanks to all of you for your support in whatever form it came.

Julia Boccumini, I am not sure I could have pulled this off without you. Thanks for the hours upon hours of dance parties, coloring, and "family." We are lucky to have you on our squad.

To my perfectly imperfect children, who inadvertently inspired a good number of the household uses in this book (see sections on: laundry, stain removal, general cleaning, air freshener, etc.), but who also unsuspectingly inspire me every single day to be a good mom and a better person: thank you, girls. I love you so much.

And finally, to my husband Mitchell: If dousing you in apple cider vinegar didn't send you running for the hills, then I guess I can't be surprised by your unfailing support, love, and encouragement even when you're sheathed in a cloud of baking soda. Still, your patience, honesty, editing, and all-around hand-holding is pivotal to my being able to pull off something like this. Thank you. For all of it. I love you.

ABOUT THE AUTHOR

Suzy Scherr, author of *The Apple Cider Vinegar Companion*, is a personal chef, writer, and culinary instructor with a knack for finding new ways to make being in the kitchen or at the table exciting, fun, and accessible. Scherr teaches, cooks for, and cooks with adults and kids, making delicious, healthy meals that utilize new products, unfamiliar ingredients, and unique ways of incorporating everyday items. Her method of cooking instruction and food education inspires confidence, creativity, and curiosity in students of all ages.

Scherr is a regular contributor to a variety of magazines and online publications including *Parents, Fit Pregnancy,* and *Every Day with Rachael Ray.* Her cooking style and passion evolved from both formal training—she has a culinary arts degree from The Institute of Culinary Education in Manhattan—as well as a lifelong obsession with food and cooking for others. Now, as a wife and mom of two young daughters, she sees even more value in the importance of seasonally fresh, simple yet inventive meals that come together in a snap.

INDEX

PHOTO CREDITS